T0385001

Melvin Delgado, PhD
Editor

# Latinos and Alcohol Use/Abuse Revisited: Advances and Challenges for Prevention and Treatment Programs

*Latinos and Alcohol Use/Abuse Revisited: Advances and Challenges for Prevention and Treatment Programs* has been co-published simultaneously as *Alcoholism Treatment Quarterly*, Volume 23, Numbers 2/3 2005.

The Haworth Press, Inc.

# Latinos and Alcohol Use/Abuse Revisited: Advances and Challenges for Prevention and Treatment Programs

*Latinos and Alcohol Use/Abuse Revisited: Advances and Challenges for Prevention and Treatment Programs* has been co-published simultaneously as *Alcoholism Treatment Quarterly*, Volume 23, Numbers 2/3 2005.

# Monographic Separates from *Alcoholism Treatment Quarterly*

For additional information on these and other Haworth Press titles, including descriptions, tables of contents, reviews, and prices, use the QuickSearch catalog at http://www.HaworthPress.com.

*Latinos and Alcohol Use/Abuse Revisited: Advances and Challenges for Prevention and Treatment Programs,* edited by Melvin Delgado, PhD (Vol. 23, No. 2/3, 2005). *"For anyone interested in building a culturally competent system of care for Latinos, This book will provide invaluable guidance. . . . Fills a substantial gap in our knowledge about alcohol use and abuse among subgroups of Latinos. . . . Brings together research and practice knowledge on a broad range of topics, including the most recent trends in alcohol use and dependence among Latinos, service use and effectiveness, help-seeking behavior and barriers to treatment, the unmet needs of incarcerated Latinos, and ethnically sensitive interventions." (Carol Coohey, PhD, Associate Professor, University of Iowa School of Social Work)*

*Responding to Physical and Sexual Abuse in Women with Alcohol and Other Drug and Mental Disorders: Program Building,* edited by Bonita M. Veysey, PhD, and Colleen Clark, PhD (Vol. 22, No. 3/4, 2004). *"Highly recommended. Any clinician working with women (and their families) will appreciate the breadth and depth of this book and its use of clinical examples, treatment direction, and sobering statistics." (John Brick, PhD, MA, FAPA, Executive Director, Intoxikon International; Author of Drugs, the Brain, and Behavior and the Handbook of the Medical Consequences of Alcohol and Drug Abuse)*

*Alcohol Problems in the United States: Twenty Years of Treatment Perspective,* edited by Thomas F. McGovern, EdD, and William L. White, MA (Vol. 20, No. 3/4, 2002). *An overview of trends in the treatment of alcohol problems over a 20-year period.*

*Homelessness Prevention in Treatment of Substance Abuse and Mental Illness: Logic Models and Implementation of Eight American Projects*, edited by Kendon J. Conrad, PhD, Michael D. Matters, PhD, Patricia Hanrahan, PhD, and Daniel J. Luchins, MD (Vol. 17, No. 1/2, 1999). *Provides you with new insights into how you can help your clients overcome political, economic, and environmental barriers to treatment that can lead to homelessness.*

*Alcohol Use/Abuse Among Latinos: Issues and Examples of Culturally Competent Services*, edited by Melvin Delgado, PhD (Vol. 16, No. 1/2, 1998). *"This book will have widespread appeal for practitioners and educators involved in direct service delivery, organizational planning, research, or policy development." (Steven Lozano Applewhite, PhD, Associate Professor, Graduate School of Social Work, University of Houston, Texas)*

*Treatment of the Addictions: Applications of Outcome Research for Clinical Management*, edited by Norman S. Miller, MD (Vol. 12, No. 2, 1994). *"Ambitious and informative . . . Recommended to anybody involved in the practice of substance abuse treatment and research in treatment outcome." (The American Journal of Addictions)*

*Self-Recovery: Treating Addictions Using Transcendental Meditation and Maharishi Ayur-Veda*, edited by David F. O'Connell, PhD, and Charles N. Alexander, PhD (Vol. 11, No. 1/2/3/4, 1994). *"A scholarly trailblazer, a scientific first. . . . Those who work daily in the fight against substance abuse, violence, and illness will surely profit from reading this important volume. A valuable new tool in what may be America's most difficult battle." (Joseph Drew, PhD, Chair for Evaluation, Mayor's Advisory Committee on Drug Abuse, Washington, DC; Professor of Political Science, University of the District of Columbia)*

*Treatment of the Chemically Dependent Homeless: Theory and Implementation in Fourteen American Projects*, edited by Kendon J. Conrad, PhD, Cheryl I. Hultman, PhD, and John S. Lyons, PhD (Vol. 10, No. 3/4, 1993). *"A wealth of information and experience. . . . A very useful reference book for everyone seeking to develop their own treatment strategies with this patient group or the homeless mentally ill." (British Journal of Psychiatry)*

*Treating Alcoholism and Drug Abuse Among Homeless Men and Women: Nine Community Demonstration Grants*, edited by Milton Argeriou, PhD, and Dennis McCarty, PhD (Vol. 7, No. 1, 1990). *"Recommended to those in the process of trying to better serve chemically dependent homeless persons." (Journal of Psychoactive Drugs)*

***Co-Dependency: Issues in Treatment and Recovery***, edited by Bruce Carruth, PhD, and Warner Mendenhall, PhD (Vol. 6, No. 1, 1989). *"At last a book for clinicians that clearly defines co-dependency and gives helpful treatment approaches. Essential."* *(Margot Escott, MSW, Social Worker in Private Practice, Naples, Florida)*

***The Treatment of Shame and Guilt in Alcoholism Counseling***, edited by Ronald T. Potter-Efron, MSW, PhD, and Patricia S. Potter-Efron, MS, CACD III (Vol. 4, No. 2, 1989). *"Comprehensive in its coverage and provides important insights into the treatment of alcoholism, especially the importance to the recovery process of working through feelings of overwhelming shame and guilt. Recommended as required reading."* *(Australian Psychologist)*

***Drunk Driving in America: Strategies and Approaches to Treatment***, edited by Stephen K. Valle, ScD, CAC, FACATA (Vol. 3, No. 2, 1986). *Creative and thought-provoking methods related to research, policy, and treatment of the drunk driver.*

***Alcohol Interventions: Historical and Sociocultural Approaches***, edited by David L. Strug, PhD, S. Priyadarsini, PhD, and Merton M. Hyman (Supp. #1, 1986). *"A comprehensive and unique account of addictions treatment of centuries ago."* *(Federal Probation: A Journal of Correctional Philosophy)*

***Treatment of Black Alcoholics***, edited by Frances Larry Brisbane, PhD, MSW, and Maxine Womble, MA (Vol. 2, No. 3/4, 1985). *"Outstanding! In view of the paucity of research on the topic, this text presents some of the outstanding work done in this area."* *(Dr. Edward R. Smith, Department of Educational Psychology, University of Wisconsin-Milwaukee)*

***Psychosocial Issues in the Treatment of Alcoholism***, edited by David Cook, CSW, Christine Fewell, ACSW, and Shulamith Lala Ashenberg Straussner, DSW, CEAP (Vol. 2, No. 1, 1985). *"Well-written and informative; the topic areas are relevant to today's social issues and offer some new approaches to the treatment of alcoholics."* *(The American Journal of Occupational Therapy)*

***Alcoholism and Sexual Dysfunction: Issues in Clinical Management***, edited by David J. Powell, PhD (Vol. 1, No. 3, 1984). *"It does a good job of explicating the linkage between two of the most common health problems in the U.S. today."* *(Journal of Sex & Marital Therapy)*

# Latinos and Alcohol Use/Abuse Revisited: Advances and Challenges for Prevention and Treatment Programs

Melvin Delgado, PhD
Editor

*Latinos and Alcohol Use/Abuse Revisited: Advances and Challenges for Prevention and Treatment Programs* has been co-published simultaneously as *Alcoholism Treatment Quarterly*, Volume 23, Numbers 2/3 2005.

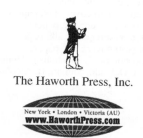

The Haworth Press, Inc.

New York • London • Victoria (AU)
www.HaworthPress.com

*Latinos and Alcohol Use/Abuse Revisited: Advances and Challenges for Prevention and Treatment Programs* has been co-published simultaneously as *Alcoholism Treatment Quarterly*, Volume 23, Numbers 2/3 2005.

The development, preparation, and publication of this work has been undertaken with great care. However, the publisher, employees, editors, and agents of The Haworth Press and all imprints of The Haworth Press, Inc., including The Haworth Medical Press® and Pharmaceutical Products Press®, are not responsible for any errors contained herein or for consequences that may ensue from use of materials or information contained in this work. Opinions expressed by the author(s) are not necessarily those of The Haworth Press, Inc. With regard to case studies, identities and circumstances of individuals discussed herein have been changed to protect confidentiality. Any resemblance to actual persons, living or dead, is entirely coincidental.

The Haworth Press, Inc., 10 Alice Street, Binghamton, 13904-1580 USA

Cover design by Lora Wiggins

**Library of Congress Cataloging-in-Publication Data**

Latinos and alcohol use/abuse revisited : advances and challenges for prevention and treatment programs / Melvin Delgado, editor.
     p. cm.
  "Co-published simultaneously as Alcoholism treatment quarterly, volume 23, numbers 2/3 2005."
Includes bibliographical references and index.
ISBN-13: 978-0-7890-2925-6 (hard cover : alk. paper)
ISBN-10: 0-7890-2925-1 (hard cover : alk. paper)
ISBN-13: 978-0-7890-2926-3 (soft cover: alk. paper)
ISBN-10: 0-7890-2926-X (soft cover : alk. paper)
  1. Hispanic Americans–Alcohol use. 2. Alcoholism–United States–Prevention. 3. Alcoholism–Treatment–United States. I. Delgado, Melvin. II. Alcoholism treatment quarterly.

HV5199.5.L38 2005
362.292'7'08968073–dc22
                                                  2005006185

# Indexing, Abstracting & Website/Internet Coverage

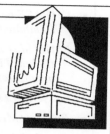

This section provides you with a list of major indexing & abstracting services and other tools for bibliographic access. That is to say, each service began covering this periodical during the year noted in the right column. Most Websites which are listed below have indicated that they will either post, disseminate, compile, archive, cite or alert their own Website users with research-based content from this work. (This list is as current as the copyright date of this publication.)

(continued)

(continued)

(continued)

*Special Bibliographic Notes related to special journal issues*
*(separates) and indexing/abstracting:*

- indexing/abstracting services in this list will also cover material in any "separate" that is co-published simultaneously with Haworth's special thematic journal issue or DocuSerial. Indexing/abstracting usually covers material at the article/chapter level.
- monographic co-editions are intended for either non-subscribers or libraries which intend to purchase a second copy for their circulating collections.
- monographic co-editions are reported to all jobbers/wholesalers/approval plans. The source journal is listed as the "series" to assist the prevention of duplicate purchasing in the same manner utilized for books-in-series.
- to facilitate user/access services all indexing/abstracting services are encouraged to utilize the co-indexing entry note indicated at the bottom of the first page of each article/chapter/contribution.
- this is intended to assist a library user of any reference tool (whether print, electronic, online, or CD-ROM) to locate the monographic version if the library has purchased this version but not a subscription to the source journal.
- individual articles/chapters in any Haworth publication are also available through the Haworth Document Delivery Service (HDDS).

# Latinos and Alcohol Use/Abuse Revisited: Advances and Challenges for Prevention and Treatment Programs

## CONTENTS

## SECTION 3: SUMMARY OF PREVENTION AND TREATMENT IMPLICATIONS

## ABOUT THE EDITOR

**Melvin Delgado, PhD,** is Professor of Social Work at Boston University School of Social Work and Graduate School of Arts and Sciences. He has published over 125 journal articles and chapters in the areas of social work in Latino communities, substance abuse prevention, natural support systems in communities of color, and social work practice with Latino elders, and has written or edited nine books. Dr. Delgado's current focus is on establishing the Boston University Social Work Minority Research Center for Research and Training in Urban Communities of Color.

# SECTION 1:
# CONTEXT SETTING
# FOR LATINOS AND ALCOHOL

## Chapter 1

# Introduction

Melvin Delgado, PhD

**SUMMARY.** The twenty-first century promises to challenge the field of alcohol research, treatment, and prevention in addressing culturally competent practice. The Latino community in the United States serves as an excellent example for measuring how far the field has progressed in meeting these challenges and identifying the work that remains to be accomplished. *[Article copies available for a fee from The Haworth Document Delivery Service: 1-800-HAWORTH. E-mail address: <docdelivery@ haworthpress.com> Website: <http://www.HaworthPress.com> © 2005 by The Haworth Press, Inc. All rights reserved.]*

**KEYWORDS.** Latinos, intervention, culture

Melvin Delgado is Professor of Social Work and Chair of Macro-Practice at Boston University School of Social Work, 264 Bay State Road, Boston, MA 02215.

Dr. Delgado wishes to acknowledge and thank the contributors of this volume who were most generous with their time and insights.

[Haworth co-indexing entry note]: "Introduction." Delgado, Melvin. Co-published simultaneously in *Alcoholism Treatment Quarterly* (The Haworth Press, Inc.) Vol. 23, No. 2/3, 2005, pp. 1-7; and: *Latinos and Alcohol Use/Abuse Revisited: Advances and Challenges for Prevention and Treatment Programs* (ed: Melvin Delgado) The Haworth Press, Inc., 2005, pp. 1-7. Single or multiple copies of this article are available for a fee from The Haworth Document Delivery Service [1-800-HAWORTH, 9:00 a.m. - 5:00 p.m. (EST). E-mail address: docdelivery@haworthpress.com].

doi:10.1300/J020v23n02_01

The field of drug abuse has received considerable national and international attention over the past twenty years. However, in this country much of this attention has focused on the role of heroin, cocaine, and crack within inner cities (Delgado, 2001; NIDA, 2003). Alcohol, with minor exceptions, has not benefited from this increased attention and funding even though its deleterious effects as measured in deaths, health problems, and financial costs are astronomical to the nation as a whole.

It has been approximately seven years since the publication of the first book that I edited entitled *Alcohol Use/Abuse Among Latinos: Issues and Examples of Culturally Competent Services*. This book was well received in the field in both scholarly and practices arenas (IDEA Prevention, 2001; Mayers, 2000; Pereira, 2000; Ruiz, 1999). This volume, like the previous one, is intended to provide an update on the latest findings and thinking on the subject of alcohol use and abuse within the Latino community in the United States, and in so doing, set the stage for what can be expected in the next decade of the twenty-first century.

This volume brings together what is arguably the most talented group of scholars on the subject and once again examines the topic from a variety of different perspectives. Each of these articles seeks to provide the reader with valuable insights into the challenges and rewards of embracing culturally competent approaches towards work in the Latino community. Every effort has been made in these articles to be specific to a particular Latino subgroup. Although it is politically advantageous to categorize all Latino subgroups into one group and label them "Latino/a," this method does a tremendous disservice to the field in better meeting their unique set of needs.

There have been dramatic changes nationally and globally since the turn of the century and millenium and this has naturally impacted on Latinos and the field of alcohol treatment services. These social, demographic, economic, political and technological changes have served to reinforce the importance and need for the field to continue its progress towards developing culturally competent research, prevention and treatment, and to do so with an understanding of the long road ahead of us (Delgado, 2002; White & McGovern, 2002).

The Latino community in the United States has continued its dramatic increase in numbers and diversity and is expected to continue to do so well into this century with Latinos having surpassed African-Americans as this nation's largest "minority" group since the latest U.S. Census Bureau counting. According to a recent Pew Hispanic Center report (Suro & Passel, 2003) the Latino population in the United States will increase from 35 million in 2000 (13 percent of all U.S. residents) to 60 million in 2020 (18 percent of all U.S. residents).

A young population and an increase in numerical representation may bring with it mixed outcomes for this community. From an advertising point of view, the Latino community in this country represents a largely untapped market. It not only has the "right" demographic picture or profile, but as a result of residential segregation, we are a market that is segmented and thus more attractive for marketers of products and services. Maxwell and Jacobson's comments over fifteen years ago are very relevant today (1989, p.ix): "Today, companies are tripping over each other in their excitement about 'discovering' the Hispanic market. They're hiring Hispanic ad agencies, advertising in Spanish-language media, and trying to forge ties with the Hispanic community by sponsoring events ranging from festivals to scholarship banquets to soccer grams. But the importance of the Hispanic market is old news for the alcohol and tobacco industries, which targeted Hispanic consumers for extensive–and profitable–advertising and promotional campaigns long before it became the fashionable thing to do."

In 2002, alcohol advertisers, for example, spent over $23 million to place advertisements in twelve or fifteen television programs favored by Latino youth (Roybal-Allard, 2003). In 1998 the top three domestic beer companies in the United States spent a combined total of almost $38 million on Latino-targeted advertisement (California-Mexico Health Initiative, 2002). Thus, increased presence and recognition brings with it increased targeting by companies. "Merchants of Death" have an uncanny ability to recognize opportunity and are not afraid to act accordingly in search of a generous profit!

Although Latinos are less likely than non-Latinos to report excessive alcohol use, Latino adolescents present a more disturbing picture. In 2000, among 12th graders, 31 percent of the Latino adolescents reported heavy drinking compared to 35 percent for white, non-Latinos (Pew Hispanic Center, 2002). They represent a potential growth market from a beer and other alcohol industry perspective with prodigious health, economic, and social consequences for this community.

This book consists of twelve chapters and is divided into three sections: (1) Context Setting for Latinos and Alcohol; (2) Prevention and Treatment; and (3) Summary of Prevention and Treatment Implications. Each of these sections is treated as their own distinct entity. However, as the reader will quickly find out, these sections and the subjects they address are highly interrelated on a daily basis in the field. The articles in this volume cover all of the major geographical sectors of this country. However, urban areas may be perceived as disproportionately represented. Nevertheless, approximately 85 to 90 percent of all Latinos residing in this country do in fact reside in urban areas.

The article by Ms. Miranda has been purposefully selected to start out the volume by providing a socio-demographic foundation, and does an excellent job of laying out Latino demographic trends and the implications they will have for the way we conceptualize the field of alcohol treatment, prevention, and research. The tremendous diversity that exists within the Latino community will manifest itself in the need for the field of alcohol services and research to be ever more specific about whom is being identified as "Latino/a" and how their socio-demographic characteristics and migration history to this country will influence service provision and eventual utilization.

Drs. Vega and Sribney have focused their expertise in better understanding the help-seeking patterns of Mexican-origin adult immigrants and Mexican-Americans living in central California. The high number of Mexican immigrants to the state of California brings with it new dynamics in how best to outreach and serve the needs of this rapidly growing population. The important role help-seeking patterns play in who and when Latinos eventually find their way into programs cannot be overly estimated.

Dr. Baez, Dr. De La Rosa and Mr. Rugh have each addressed a population that we will no doubt be in greater contact within this decade. Dr. Baez has focused on Dominican youth, a Latino group that has experienced dramatic demographic increases, particularly in New York City, within the past decade. Dominican youth bring with them many of the same issues facing their Cuban and Puerto Rican counterparts within the United States, but also bring a unique set of issues that effectively makes them substantially different from their Caribbean counterparts. Dr. De La Rosa and Mr. Rugh, in turn, present on preliminary findings from an ethnographic study of Puerto Rican/Dominican male gang members in a large New England city. The subject of gangs and the role of alcohol and other drugs has only recently started to receive the attention it deserves in the professional literature. These authors specifically focus their article on the patterns of alcohol and other drug initiation, with far ranging implications for prevention and early intervention.

This nation's prisons and jails are a testament to the role of alcohol and other drug abuse in criminal behavior (Valle & Humphrey, 2002). Dr. Garcia's article brings into focus a population group that is increasing in representation but very much overlooked in the professional literature–namely, the incarcerated Latina. Women make up the fastest growing sector of this nation's incarceration population, and Latinas make up a significant portion of this group alongside African-American women. The issues and needs of Latina inmates brings with it a set of challenges and rewards unparalleled in the field of alcohol treatment.

Dr. Bullock, too, has focused on Latinas but approached the subject from the viewpoint of caregivers–more specifically rural Latina grandmothers in a southern state. The role of grandmothers within the Latino culture is very much revered. They are often called upon to provide a wide range of expressive and instrumental care regardless of their own individual circumstances. However, they are now being thrust into roles that are unprecedented because of the impact of alcohol and other drug abuse in their families.

There are many other population subgroups, however, that have not seen a tremendous amount of attention in the professional literature. Dr. Pabon, for example, has written about Latino juvenile offenders and the importance of culture-specific programming to meet their alcohol and other drug abuse-specific needs. Latino youth within the juvenile justice system will in all likelihood eventually wind up in adult correctional systems if their unique needs are left unaddressed. This career path, so to speak, brings with it incredible implications for family structure within Latino communities. Dr. Lundgren, Capalla and Ben-Ami have focused their attention on the polydrug user, in this instance, alcohol use among Puerto Rican heroin injection drug users in a large New England city. The days of abusing just one drug seem quite distant, bringing new challenges to treating the polydrug using Latino. However, the role of alcohol in the life of heroin injection drug users is poorly understood because of common perceptions that heroin users, in this case Puerto Ricans, are primarily only interested in one drug–namely, heroin. Nevertheless, Dr. Lundgren and colleagues report on findings that will prove intriguing to the reader.

Dr. Holleran and colleagues, in turn, provide a prevention model with specific reference to alcohol and other drug use among Latino youth in the Southwest. This article uplifts the importance of an Orthogonal model of acculturation and highlights an innovative video as a method in prevention programs. The subject of acculturation and the role it plays within the Latino community has been controversial, particularly when examined within the light that newcomers to this country are far healthier than those born here or after they have been here a considerable of time. Namely, entering this country can be detrimental to your health. Dr. Holleran and colleagues shed new light on this debate.

Delgado and Rosati's article is on religion and the potential role it can have in the development of prevention and treatment programs in this field. There is general agreement in the field that natural support systems must be seriously considered in the development of any culturally competent approach towards better addressing the needs of Latinos in the United States, and religion certainly is a central component of this construct (Delgado, 1996). The authors have specifically targeted Pentecostalism because of its increased popularity within the Latino community in the United States. Finally, Delgado provides the reader with a summary and overview of the key themes and issues raised by the authors of this volume.

## *CONCLUSION*

Special issues regardless of their foci have an important place in the professional literature. They provide an editor with an unusual ability to bring together expertise that does not reside within any one individual, regardless of their abilities and wisdom. Collectively, however, individual expertise can help form a more complete picture of a complex phenomenon such as alcohol use and abuse among Latinos, and how best to provide valuable services. There is little question that special issues bring a certain focus on issues that generally get overlooked in the process of planning and delivering services in the field of alcohol and other drug abuse.

This volume has the benefits of focusing on particular group (Latinos/as). Yet, the subject matter defies limiting it to twelve articles, regardless of their breadth and the level of expertise of the authors. The reader, I believe, will be able to take many of the recommendations raised in this volume and bring them to fruition in their respective communities. I sincerely hope that the reader has as much enjoyment in reading this volume as I have had in putting it together! It is fitting to end this introduction to this volume with a quote from the Hispanic Pew Center (Suro & Passel, 2003, p.9): "Regardless of whether immigration flows from Latin America increase[s], decreases or stay the same, a great change in the composition of the Hispanic population is underway. . . . One prediction about second-generation Latinos, however, seems safe: Given their numbers, their future will be a matter of national interest."

# REFERENCES

California-Mexico Health Initiative. (2002). *Alcohol and drug consumption: Health fact sheet.* Berkeley, CA: University of California, Policy Research Center.

Delgado, M. (2002). Latinos and alcohol: Treatment considerations. *Alcoholism Treatment Quarterly,* 20, pp.187-192.

Delgado, M. (2001). *Where are all of the young men and women of color? Capacity enhancement practice and the criminal justice system.* New York: Columbia University Press.

Delgado, M. (1996). Puerto Rican natural support systems and the field of AOD: Implications for religious institutions. *Journal of Ministry in Addiction & Recovery,* 3, pp.67-77.

*IDEA Prevention.* (1998). Book Review. Author, 17, p.105.

Maxwell, B. & Jacobson, M. (1989). *Marketing disease to Hispanics: The selling of alcohol, tobacco, and junk foods.* Washington, D.C.: Center for Science in the Public Interest.

Mayers, R.S. (2000). Book Review. *Journal of Ethnic & Cultural Diversity in Social Work,* 9, pp.158-160.

National Institute of Drug Abuse. (2003). *Drug use among racial/ethnic minorities.* Rockville, MD: Author.

Pereira, J. (2002). Book review of alcohol use among Latinos: Issues and examples of culturally competent services. Edited by Melvin Delgado. *Journal of Social Work Practice in the Addictions,* 2, pp.148-149.

Pew Hispanic Center. (2002). *Hispanic health: Divergent and changing.* Washington, D.C.: Author.

Roybal-Allard, L. (2003). Cinco de Mayo. (http:www.house.gov/royal-allard/press/oped-cincodemayo.htm).

Ruiz, P. (1999). Book review of alcohol use among Latinos: Issues and examples of culturally competent services. *Transcultural Psychiatry Newsletter,* January, p.10.

Suro, R. & Passel, J.S. (2003). *The rise of the second generation: Changing patterns in Hispanic population growth.* Washington, D.C.: Pew Hispanic Center.

Valle, S.K. & Humphrey, D. (2002). American prisons as alcohol and drug treatment centers: A twenty-year reflection, 1980 to 2000. *Alcohol Treatment Quarterly,* 20, pp.83-106.

White, W.L. & McGovern, T.F. (2002). Treating alcohol problems: A future perspective. *Alcoholism Treatment Quarterly,* 20, pp.233-239.

Chapter 2

# Brief Overview of Latino Demographics in the Twenty-First Century: Implications for Alcohol-Related Services

Celina Miranda, MSW, MEd

**SUMMARY.** The Latino population in the United States has grown substantially in the past twenty years. It is expected that by the year 2050, Latinos will comprise twenty-four percent of the total U.S. population. The growth of the Latino population poses many challenges for alcohol-related services. The increasing diversity of the population changes the framework for culturally competent services. *[Article copies available for a fee from The Haworth Document Delivery Service: 1-800-HAWORTH. E-mail address: <docdelivery@haworthpress.com> Website: <http://www.HaworthPress. com> © 2005 by The Haworth Press, Inc. All rights reserved.]*

**KEYWORDS.** Latinos, demographics, alcohol, services

## INTRODUCTION

At the turn of the twenty-first century, Latinos became the largest minority group in the United States. The 2000 Census reported that the La-

Celina Miranda is a doctoral student at Boston University School of Graduate Studies in the joint degree program in social work and sociology.

[Haworth co-indexing entry note]: "Brief Overview of Latino Demographics in the Twenty-First Century: Implications for Alcohol-Related Services." Miranda, Celina. Co-published simultaneously in *Alcoholism Treatment Quarterly* (The Haworth Press, Inc.) Vol. 23, No. 2/3, 2005, pp. 9-27; and: *Latinos and Alcohol Use/Abuse Revisited: Advances and Challenges for Prevention and Treatment Programs* (ed: Melvin Delgado) The Haworth Press, Inc., 2005, pp. 9-27. Single or multiple copies of this article are available for a fee from The Haworth Document Delivery Service [1-800-HAWORTH, 9:00 a.m. - 5:00 p.m. (EST). E-mail address: docdelivery@haworthpress.com].

Available online at http://www.haworthpress.com/web/ATQ
© 2005 by The Haworth Press, Inc. All rights reserved.
doi:10.1300/J020v23n02_02

tino population at 35.3 million had surpassed the African American population of 34.7 million (U.S. Bureau of the Census, 2000). In the past twenty years (1980-2000), the Latino population has grown substantially. This rapid growth is expected to continue throughout this century. Encapsulating the Latino population in a succinct overview is challenging due to the growing complexity of this population. The Latino population is exceptionally diverse. By no accounts has this population ever been homogeneous; however, the population's growing diversity is becoming more visible today. The three traditional Latino groups–Mexican, Puerto Rican, and Cuban–have recently been joined by an influx of immigrants and refugees from all parts of Latin America and the Spanish-speaking Caribbean.

Immigration has commonly been considered an urban phenomenon concentrated in the largest cities (Portes & Rumbaut, 1996). Latinos are more likely to live in metropolitan areas than the general population. In 2000, of the largest cities in the U.S. only two, Detroit and Philadelphia, were less than one-quarter Latino (Population Resource Center, 2002). However, in recent years there has been a spreading-out effect from rural and urban to suburban areas (Cohn, July 31, 2003; Population Resource Center, 2002a). An increasing number of Latino immigrants are bypassing the central cities in hopes of better job opportunities and setting root in non-traditional geographic destinations.

The purpose of this chapter is to provide a brief overview of Latino demographics in the twenty-first century and the implications for alcohol-related services. As stated earlier, a concise summary is challenging because of the current reality of Latinos in this country at the turn of this century. Issues of legal status; family composition; first, second, and third generation identification; national origin and identity; age; and others arise as one begins to make sense of this broadly defined population. The reader should use caution in drawing generalizations from the data provided in this overview. Instead, this overview should be used to set the context as we expand and enhance culturally competent alcohol-related services for Latinos in the United States. Issues and challenges to culturally appropriate ATOD services for Latinos have been addressed in the literature (Delgado, 1997; Rodriguez-Andrew, 1998; Paz, 2002); however, in the twenty-first century the framework for offering culturally competent services to Latinos has become more complex.

## LATINO OR HISPANIC?

Before moving forward, the terms "Latino" and "Hispanic" need to be briefly discussed. Latinos is used to refer to the U.S. population that traces its descent back to the Spanish-speaking Caribbean and other parts of Latin America (Suárez-Orozco & Páez, 2002). The term Latino gained popularity in the 1990s (Mayo-Quiñones & Helfgot, 2003) and is preferred over the term Hispanic by some. Although the federal government in the 1970s adopted the term Hispanic, the term Latino is seen as more inclusive of the indigenous and African cultures of Latin America (Flores cited in Timmins, 2002). This chapter will continue to use the term Latino in referring to this population.

Collapsing subgroups into one all-encompassing term can be seen as simultaneously problematic and beneficial. To this point Hero (1992) states, "(. . .) individual and group identifications may serve purposes of pride and self-esteem: self-identification may also serve 'strategic' purposes, leading to greater access to government programs and benefits" (p. 4). In addition, as a visibly expanding group, Latinos have been able to gain political visibility as is reflected by political candidates' efforts to reach Spanish-speaking segments of the U.S. population in recent years. Suárez-Orozco and Páez (2002) further argue that scholarly reflection at the panethnic level can also be expressed from a standpoint of theoretical considerations rather than politics. They state, "work at the panethnic level can generate more robust conceptual understandings than work at the subgroup level" (p. 6). Moreover, there are research advantages for reporting findings under one heading; however, this practice has resulted in difficulties in understanding alcohol use among Latino subgroups (Rodriguez-Andrew, 1998). In the latter argument Rodriguez-Andrew (1998) agrees with Suárez-Orozco and Páez (2002); however, she also emphasizes that in order to improve services we need to learn more about substance abuse at the subgroup level.

## A PROFILE OF THE LATINO POPULATION

From 1980 to 2000, the Latino population more than doubled from 14.6 million to 35.3 million (Hobbs & Stoops, 2002). This demographic growth trend is expected to continue for decades to come. From April 2000 to July 2002 alone, the Latino population saw an increase of 3.5 million raising the Latino population to over 38 million (Wall, June 19, 2003). According to the U.S. Census middle series projections, the percentage of Latinos in the total population could rise from 12.5 percent in 2000 to 24 percent in 2050 (Guzmán, 2001; Hollman & Mulder, January 13, 2000). The substantial growth in the past twenty years of the Latino population can be attributed to high immigration and birth rates (Vega, 1990; Mayo-Quiñones & Helfgot, 2003; Kitty & Haynes, 2000). It is posited that the Latino population is more numerous than reported in the Census, once the estimated five to eight million undocumented immigrants are added to official counts (Wall, June 19, 2003).

## The New Immigration

Immigration in the past twenty years has accounted for more than a third of the total population growth in the United States. Asian and Latino populations grew particularly in both absolute and relative size (Zhou, 2002). Much of the observed growth of the Latino population is accounted to high immigration rates. Scholars typically divide the history of U.S. immigration into three phases: 1901 to 1930, classic era of European immigration; 1931 to 1970, a long hiatus of limited movement; and 1970 to the present, non-European immigration (Massey, 1995). Latinos from all over Latin America and the Caribbean are largely found in the new immigration of non-Europeans. According to the 2002 Current Population Report, Latinos accounted for 52.2 percent of the total foreign-born population (Schmidley, 2003). In 1997, Mexico alone made up 7.0 million of the total foreign born compared to 800,000 in 1970, while Cuba, the Dominican Republic, and El Salvador were among the top ten countries of birth of the foreign born (Census Brief: Coming to America, 2000).

Several policies have been developed in the past twenty years to curtail immigration, especially illegal immigration. The 1980 Refugee Act broadened the definition of political refugee by adopting United Nations definitions (Kilty & Vidal de Haymes, 2000). This opened the door for political refugees from various Latin American countries to seek entry into the United States. However, there are restrictions as to how many refugees can be accepted each year, which has raised concern over illegal entrance. In addition, the 1986 Immigration and Reform Control Act (IRCA) was responsible for the legalization of over 3.3 million former undocumented migrants (Massey, 1995). Of those legalized under IRCA, 75 percent were Mexican (Massey, 1995). In order to reduce illegal immigration, IRCA proposed two things: (1) granting amnesty to current undocumented immigrants living in the U.S. and (2) imposing sanctions on employers who hired "illegals" in the future (Kilty & Vidal de Haymes, 2000).

These measures have been unsuccessful in discouraging illegal immigration and in 1997, the illegal population was estimated at over five million (Martin & Midgley cited in Kilty & Vidal de Haymes, 2000). Kilty and Vidal de Haymes (2000) point to the latest federal effort to reduce illegal immigration, which was in 1996, the Illegal Immigration Reform and Immigration Responsibility Act. This legislation created more punitive provisions than the earlier legislation of 1986 (Kilty & Vidal de Haymes, 2000). Legality issues are a concern for many recent immigrants. Particular policies have benefited certain groups such as NACARA (Nicaraguan Adjustment and Central American Relief Act) and TPS (temporary protected status), which apply to individuals from El Salvador, Honduras, and Nicaragua. Furthermore, arrival to this country either as a refugee, legal immigrant, or undocumented immigrant raises issues of family and family reunification. Zhou (2002) states that admission of refugees implies an enlarged base for future immigration due to family reunification. Continuing immigration, both legal and illegal, will indisputably remain a high source of the projected population growth for Latinos.

### Growing Population Diversity

Mexicans continue to be the largest Latino subgroup in the United States. In 2000, among the Latino population 58.5 percent were Mexican, 9.6 percent were Puerto Rican, 4.8 percent were Central American, 3.8 percent were South American, 3.5 percent were Cuban, and 17.3 percent were other Hispanic (Guzmán, 2001). The "other Hispanic" category experienced a 96.9 percent increase from 5.1 million in 1990 to 10.0 million in 2000 (Guzmán, 2001). The unprecedented increase of the "other Hispanic" population sparked controversy among representatives of several national origin groups who felt their communities were undercounted (Suro, 2002). Consequently, an alternative estimate of the breakdown of the Hispanic population by national origin has been calculated in a report published by the Pew Hispanic Center using Census 2000 Supplementary Survey data. These estimates reduced the "other" category by more than half and did not alter the overall size of the population (Suro, 2002). According to these estimates, the Dominican population is approximately 938,316 individuals compared to the 764,945 reported in the Census 2000, a 22.7 percent difference. Salvadorans are estimated to be 958,487 compared to 655,165 in the

Census 2000, a 46.3 percent difference, while Guatemalans were estimated at, 534,951 compared to 372,487 according to the 2000 Census, a 43.6 percent difference. Overall, estimates presented in the report indicate that the Census 2000 overestimated the preference to identify under the all-encompassing "other Hispanic" label and underestimated specific nationality identification. Estimates in Suro (2002) are extremely important and should not be ignored. Primarily, these estimates give a more accurate portrayal of the subgroup diversification that has taken place in the past few decades. The growing diversity of Latinos must be acknowledged as social interventions are pushed forward at both the national and community level.

Immigration only accounts for part of the Latino population growth in the past twenty years. Second and third generation Latinos have also contributed to the population expansion. In the span of thirty years (1970 to 2000), the Latino population grew by 25.7 million. Immigrants accounted for 45 percent of that increase while the second generation accounted for 28 percent and the third generation accounted for 27% (Suro & Passel, 2003). Suro and Passel (2003) estimate that the Latino population will grow by 25 million between 2000 and 2020; in that time period, the Latino second generation is estimated to account for 47 percent of the increase to 25 percent for the first. They also estimate that by the year 2020, the second generation will outnumber the first generation. Latino population growth will be affected not only by continuing immigration, but also by increasing second and third generation births.

The diversification of the Latino population therefore extends beyond subgroup identity. Population needs shift as they become more entrenched in this country through acculturation processes. Appropriate social services for a recent immigrant are drastically different from those needed by a second or third generation immigrant. As a result, in designing culturally competent ATOD services several factors need to be considered.

### Geographic Concentration of Latinos

Latinos can be found throughout the country with some geographic areas having larger concentrations. According to the 2000 Census, 43.5 percent of Latinos live in the West and 32.8 percent live in the South. Meanwhile, the Northeast and Midwest accounted for 14.9 and 8.9 percent respectively (Guzmán, 2001). Nearly half (46.4%) of all Latinos in 2000 lived in a central city within a metropolitan area compared with slightly more than one-fifth (21.2%) of non-Hispanic

Whites (Therrien & Ramirez, 2001). Over half of Latinos live in two states, California (11.0 million) and Texas (6.7 million). New York (2.9 million), Florida (2.7 million), Illinois (1.5 million), Arizona (1.3 million), and New Jersey (1.1 million) have Latino populations of one million or more (Population Resource Center, 2002).

Latinos continue to be highly concentrated in certain areas of the country. However, the past ten years has seen an increase of Latinos in parts of the country where few were present in the past. Cohn (July 31, 2003) states that areas that once had small Latino populations have experienced tremendous growth rates in recent years. For instance, the Washington area (stretching from Southern Maryland to West Virginia) Latino population has risen by 336 percent in the last two decades (Cohn, July 31, 2003), while North Carolina has seen a 394 percent increase in its Latino population in the past ten years (Kitchen, 2002). Moreover, the Latino population grew by 995 percent in Atlanta, 962 percent in Charlotte, and 859 percent in Orlando (Population Resource Center, 2002). Latino immigrants are avoiding the usual metropolitan receiving cities for places where there are more jobs. This current demographic change raises concerns over accessibility and availability to meet the needs of the growing Latino population in these communities.

## Age

Latinos are a young population. A large percent of Latinos are younger than 18 years of age. According to Therrien and Ramirez (2001) in 2000, 35.7 percent of the Latino population was younger than 18 years of age compared with 23.5 percent for non-Hispanic Whites. Of the various Latino subgroups, Mexicans had the highest proportion of population under 18 years of age at 38.4 percent compared with Cubans who had the lowest at 19.2 percent (Therrien & Ramirez, 2001). A relatively small percent (5.3) of the Latino population was 65 and older compared with non-Hispanic Whites (14.0 percent). Meanwhile, 32.4 percent of the Latino population was between the ages of 25 to 44 compared to 29.5 percent for the non-Hispanic White population (Therrien & Ramirez, 2001).

## Poverty

Poverty is one of the most serious problems affecting the Latino population in the United States (De La Rosa, 2000). In 2001, the poverty rate for Latinos was 21.4 percent compared to 22.7 percent for Blacks and 7.8 percent for non-Hispanic Whites (Proctor & Delaker, September 2002). Although the poverty rates for Latinos did not change between 2000 and 2001, the number of poor Latinos rose from 7.7 million in 2000 to 8.0 million in 2001 (Proctor & Delaker, September 2002). De La Rosa (2000) points out that many Latino families live in poverty. In 2001, 19.4 percent of Latino families lived below the poverty level compared to 5.7 percent of non-Hispanic White families. Family composition affects Latino poverty. For Latino married couples in 2001, 13.8 percent live below the poverty level compared to 3.3 percent for non-Hispanic Whites (Proctor & Delaker, September 2002). As pointed out by De La Rosa (2000), the poverty rates for families headed by single females are astoundingly high. In 2001, the percent of Latino families headed by single females living below the poverty level rose slightly from 36.4 in 2000 to 37.0 in 2001 (Proctor & Delaker, September 2002). For Latino children and adolescents ages 18 and younger, 28.0 percent were living in poverty in 2001 compared 9.5 percent for non-Hispanic Whites (Proctor & Delaker, September 2002). Poverty continues to disproportionately affect Latinos in this country.

### Education

Latinos have relatively low levels of educational attainment. Some scholars have made a direct connection between low educational attainment among Latinos and poverty levels of this population (De La Rosa, 2000). According to the March 2002 Current Population Survey, out of Latinos aged 25 and over, 57.0 percent had completed four years of high school or more compared to 88.7 for non-Hispanic Whites (U.S. Census Bureau, 2003). Latinos born in the United States were more likely to have a bachelor's degree (14 percent) compared to Latinos born outside of the country (9 percent) (U.S. Census Bureau, 2003). According to the Census Current Population Survey March 2000, Cubans (73.0 percent) and other Latinos (71.6 percent) were more likely to have graduated from high school than Mexicans (51.0 percent) (Therrien & Ramirez, 2001).

### LATINO ALCOHOL USE/ABUSE

There is intragroup variation in Latino alcohol use patterns. Current demographic trends of the Latino population, particularly its growing diversity, necessitates for research to continue to add to our understanding while keeping in mind the complex nature of this population in this country. Alcohol use patterns need to be examined not simply for Latinos as a whole group, but also by specific national identity as one example. How do drinking patterns vary for Guatemalans compared to Puerto Ricans in the U.S.? Other covariates such as level of acculturation, gender, generation in the U.S., and age need to be included in future research designs. Recent literature on alcohol and other drugs is showing progress in this direction by moving beyond the homogeneous grouping of Latinos and looking specifically at Cuban, Mexican, Puerto Rican, and other Latino subgroups (Kail, Zayas, & Malgady, 2000; Nielsen, 2000; Nielsen, 2001; Khoury et al., 1996). Findings indicate that there are significant differences between subgroups. Current research however has not kept up with subgroups such as Salvadorans, Colombians, and Guatemalans, which represent immigrants that are more recent to this country. The purpose of this section is not to present a thorough overview of the literature on Latino alcohol use and abuse. Rather it will highlight recent findings and conclude with research implications based on these findings.

A recent publication by the National Institute on Drug Abuse (2003) points to variations of drug use among the Latino population. National Household Survey on Drug Abuse (NHSDA) combined data for 1997 and 1998 indicates that 52.4 percent of 26- to 34-year-old Latinos reported alcohol use in the past month, compared to 49.7 percent for 18 to 25, 45.3 percent for 35 and over, and 18.9 for those ages 12 to 17 (NIDA, 2003). Those who identified as South American (66.5%) between 18 and 25 had a greater percent of reported alcohol use in the past month than Puerto Rican (54.1%), Mexican (47.7%), Cuban (47.9%), Central American (53.2 %), and other (52.1%) of the same age group.

Moreover, Latinas reported lower alcohol use in the past month than the men (55.2 and 32.2 percent respectively) (NIDA, 2003), while Mexicans (7.4 percent) were more likely to report heavy alcohol use (5 or more drinks on the same occasion on at least 5 or more days prior to assessment) followed by Puerto Ricans (6.4 percent), Central Americans (4.1 percent), South Americans (4.1 percent), others (3.2 percent), and Cubans (1.7 percent) (NIDA, 2003). However, when broken down by age group, South Americans (17.2 percent), Puerto Ricans (11.9 percent), and Central Americans (10.7 percent) ages 18 to 25 reported the higher percentages of heavy alcohol use in the past month. In addition, South American youth ages 12 to 17 were more likely to report alcohol use in the past month (23.9 percent) and heavy alcohol use (11.4 percent) (NIDA, 2003).

Looking at drinking patterns among ethnic groups by age and gender, Neilsen (2000) found that "other Hispanics" are significantly less likely than Mexican Americans to drink. The "other Hispanic" referred to respondents who did not identify as Mexican, Cuban, or Puerto Rican. Moreover, among respondents who drink, Cubans and "other Hispanics" are significantly less likely than Mexican Americans to be frequent high maximum and heavy drinkers (Neilsen, 2000). In another study, Neilsen (2001) looked at adult roles and their effect on drinking patterns for Mexicans, Cubans, Puerto Ricans, other Latinos, and Whites. Findings indicate that Cuban parents are less likely to drink than are respondents with no children. Moreover, for all ethnic groups except for Cubans, married persons are less likely to drink heavily than single or divorced/separated respondents. Looking at problems experienced due to heavy drinking, Neilsen (2001) also found variation among the ethnic groups. For Whites, Cubans, and Puerto Ricans married persons are less likely to experience problems than are non-married people. For other Latinos, married persons are more likely than are non-married people to have problems. Mexicans did not significantly differ by marital status (Neilsen, 2001).

Intragroup variation was also found in a study by Kail, Zayas and Malgady (2000), which examined differences among Colombian, Dominican, and Puerto Rican men in regard to motivations for drinking and how these motivations, depressive symptomatology, and acculturation are related to frequency and quantity of drinking. Among several findings, they found that Puerto Ricans showed higher levels of acculturation than the other two groups. Moreover, for Puerto Ricans, acculturation and depression seemed to predict psychological motivations for drinking, while for Dominican men, depression seemed to predict drinking for psychological reasons. For Colombian men, depression appears to predict psychological motivations for drinking. These findings need to be interpreted cautiously due to methodological considerations due to nonrandom sampling. Nevertheless, these findings point to significant differences in the motivations for drinking among these Latino subgroups that should not be overlooked and need further study.

Culturally competent alcohol-related services are contingent on growing understanding of Latino alcohol use in the context of the population's social, cultural, and historical experience in this country. Vega, Gil, and Kolody (2002) argue that though difficult to predict, current demographic trends will influence drug-use patterns for Latinos (Vega, Gil, & Kolody, 2002). Among these demographic trends is the growing geographic dispersal of Latinos throughout the country. They further state that a weakness of large surveys that gather data on Latino drug use is the failure to distinguish nationality or birthplace subgroups (Vega, Gil, & Kolody, 2002). Moreover, Kail, Zayas and Malgady (2000) argue that it is essential to designing culturally competent interventions to continue to increase the knowledge on the intracultural variations, antecedents, and outcomes of alcohol use. There is overwhelming agreement in the literature that research needs to continue its focus on subgroups' particular alcohol use patterns to better understand the issue for Latinos in the United States (Vega, Gil, & Kolody, 2002; Kail, Zayas, & Malgady, 2000; Neilsen, 2001).

Research looking at alcohol use within the Latino population needs to continue gaining sophistication and rigor as it controls for compounding variables that have generally been overlooked. These variables include and are not limited to age, gender, years in the U.S., income, acculturation, and generation. In addition, other research needs to look at use by type of alcohol and its sociohistorical role for particular subgroups. For instance, Delgado (1997) states that historically alcohol has been used as a tool of social control, in particular among low-skilled workers. Rum in places such as the Dominican Republic, Puerto Rico, and Cuba, for instance, has been and continues to be relatively inexpensive (Delgado, 1997). Does the sociopolitical and historical context of rum continue to affect the use of this particular type of alcohol for these subpopulations in the United States? Furthermore, increasing the knowledge base can help inform providers as they seek to design culturally appropriate alcohol-related services. Only through collaboration with community-based agencies and natural support systems (see Delgado, 1998) can research keep pace with the growing diversity of Latinos. Communities where emerging groups are relocating can serve as hubs for groundbreaking research, given that communities have greater venues for access to emerging populations that otherwise are hard to reach. Therefore, it is essential to continuously narrow the gap between research and communities to enhance our understanding of alcohol use among all Latinos in this country.

## CHALLENGES TO INTERPRETING DEMOGRAPHIC DATA

Interpreting demographic data presents several challenges. Although this discussion is most likely not being presented to the reader for the first time, the writer deems it necessary to briefly discuss few of these presenting challenges in this section. Varied data sources and methodological issues need to be kept in mind when interpreting data. For instance, the Census 2000 form changed from that used in 1990, in particular the question to determine Latino heritage changed in wording (Suro, 2002). This minor change had several implications for analysis. At first glance, the data indicated that Latinos were increasingly less likely to report their national identity and instead select "other Hispanic." As discussed earlier, a closer look at the methods showed that seemingly minor word changes from one data point to the next may have had a large effect on this observed difference.

Relying on census data presents additional challenges for interpretation. Census data are expressed data and therefore have several limitations. The data are cross-sectional in nature, which means that they capture only one point in time. Consequently, the picture painted by demographic data should be cautiously interpreted and presented. Undoubtedly the data misses a whole section of the population who either by choice or fear of deportation decides not to fill out forms. Undocumented populations along with other vulnerable groups (e.g., poor and homeless) are indisputably undercounted in demographic counts. Moreover, these data do not account for transient populations. Latino migrant workers and others with high mobility rates may also be undercounted or missed all together. Finally, demographic data are recorded by formal institutional settings. These settings may have limited access to emerging populations due to institutional barriers. As a result, these institutions may not have the full picture that local and community-based organizations informally are able to record. The portrait of Latinos in the United States presented through the use of demographic data needs to be interpreted carefully while accounting for its many limitations.

## IMPLICATIONS FOR ALCOHOL-RELATED SERVICES

Shifting Latino demographics in the twenty-first century have a series of implications for alcohol-related services. The portrait of this population is rapidly changing. As Delgado (2002) points out, for instance, communities that were historically Mexican are being transformed by a combination of groups from Central and South America. These transformations are taking place throughout the country. In addition, continuous immigration from all over Latin America raises concerns over accessibility of social services. Accessibility to social services is restricted for this population due to language, cultural, and economic barriers. As stated previously, the literature has addressed the need for culturally competent alcohol services for Latinos. However, it can be argued that the Latino population is at a defining moment at the break of this new century and, consequently, there is an open opportunity to enhance previous frameworks for culturally competent services in this context. The following section will outline some of the key implications for alcohol-related services that have surfaced from the present overview.

## Legal Status

Legal status has critical implications for the provision of alcohol-related services for the Latino population. Not all subgroups are affected the same way. Puerto Ricans, for instance, do not have to be concerned over their immigration status given they are citizens of the United States. Delgado (1998) points out that, "The fact that Puerto Ricans are United States citizens presents a different challenge to service delivery compared with Hispanics who are in the United States with an undocumented status" (p. 90). For individuals that enter the country undocumented, their legal status in itself becomes one more barrier to accessing services. Delgado (2002) states, "The documented status of Latinos wield a tremendous amount of influence in dictating the help-seeking patterns they can safely exercise in this country" (p. 190). The fear of deportation can be a primary deterrent to accessing social services when available for illegal immigrants or family members without legal status (Strug & Mason, 2002).

Upon arriving to the country, immigrants are not immune to negative social conditions. "Whether immigrants, refugees, or asylum seekers, displaced persons become migrants who suffer a number of social conditions which make them vulnerable, thus often requiring the help of care-givers" (Martínez-Brawley & Zorita, 2001, p. 51). Among these social conditions of course is the abuse of alcohol and related problems. Martínez-Brawley and Zorita (2001) further point out that the government does not fund programs or services for undocumented immigrants or asylum seekers other than emergency medical care. Therefore, illegal immigrants are left to the care of organizations that rely on non-governmental funding to meet their needs (Martínez-Brawley & Zorita, 2001). Illegal Latino immigrants face greater vulnerability and marginalization due to limited levels of support available for this population. Barriers of accessibility (e.g., language, culture) are compounded by the reality that at times services needed by undocumented immigrants may not be available in some communities.

Providers of alcohol-related services need to be in tune with legal issues of the Latino population. Strug and Mason (2002) note that legal status can be a barrier to service utilization. In this respect, providers need to educate the targeted population on qualification criteria for services. Furthermore, it is important for immigrants to feel welcome in social service agencies. Strug and Mason (2002) point out that language barriers and previous experiences of discrimination can further isolate illegal immigrants and keep them from seeking services when needed. Legal status issues as well as culturally appropriateness of services must be kept in mind both during the planning and implementation stages of alcohol-related services.

### *Family*

Family can play an important role in alcohol-related services. The incorporation of family into services however raises several concerns. Primarily, family defined strictly as immediate members (e.g., mother, father, and children) is restrictive in this case. It is too limiting and fails in capturing other individuals that may be considered family or "like family" for Latino subgroups. In discussing natural support systems, Delgado (1998) argues that family needs to be defined broadly incorporating blood relatives, relatives by marriage, close family friends, and special neighbors. Neighbors and friends are especially important when talking about people that have recently arrived to the United States. Oftentimes immigration takes place one family member at a time. Other times, the stay in this country is seen as temporary usually for financial reasons. Consequently until family members arrive or during their stay in the country, these individuals often turn to neighbors and close friends for support and treat them "like family." Moreover, reunification of family is oftentimes constrained by legal issues, financial means, and immigration restrictions. Therefore, interventions will more appropriately meet the needs of Latino subgroups by espousing a broader definition of family.

This in turn requires changes in the organization. One reflection of meaningful change can be seen in respective assessment forms. Forms should reflect a broader conceptualization of family. Rather than placing the burden on the one seeking services, organizations need to take that first step and ask the appropriate questions that show receptivity to including friends and neighbors as part of the family unit. Overall, family can play a key role in alcohol-related services; however, family narrowly defined can also become a deterrent to accessing services.

## *Communities*

Communities are in constant transition. Key demographic trends show that the growing diversity of the Latino population is remarkably affecting many communities throughout the United States. Communities that previously had small number of Latinos have in recent years experienced overwhelming growth. This has been the case for Orlando, Atlanta and Charlotte, for instance, which in the past years have experienced an over 900 percent increase in their Latino population (Population Resource Center, 2002). The dispersal of Latinos throughout various parts of the country however is not the only change communities are experiencing. Communities that historically for the most part have been made up of one specific group such as Puerto Rican, Cuban, or Mexican are being transformed as other Latinos are setting roots in these communities (Delgado, 2002). These new configurations of Latinos in one community have important implications for alcohol-related services. For instance, services deemed culturally appropriate for Dominicans are not necessarily appropriate for recent immigrants from Colombia.

The changes communities are undergoing have serious implications for the accessibility of alcohol-related services. Delgado (2002) states that accessibility to alcohol-related services for Latinos in this country requires that organization address four key arenas. The first is *geographical accessibility*, which refers to the location of services. The second arena is *psychological accessibility*, referring to comfort level Latinos experience in accessing social services. The third and fourth arenas are *cultural* and *operational accessibility*. Cultural accessibility refers to organizations that use the language of preference, cultural traditions, staffing with similar ethnic/cultural heritage as the consumer, and understanding of cultural values and beliefs, while operational accessibility refers to the hours of operation (Delgado, 2002).

Psychological accessibility and cultural accessibility are key arenas that need to be addressed in communities where the composition of Latinos is changing. Strug and Mason (2002), for example, point out that in Washington Heights most community-based organizations were established to meet the needs of the Dominican population, which has left the growing Guatemalan, Honduran, and Mexican populations with limited choices for services. This example can be applied to other areas where these reconfigurations of the Latino population are taking place.

Organizations that have been set up to meet one particular Latino sub-group need to deal with all four areas of accessibility, especially the arenas of psychological and cultural accessibility. New communities' members need to feel welcome in the existing organizations so that they can access existing social services. Moreover, the organizations need to be trained in the cultural values and beliefs of the new groups joining the community. The assumption that Latinos are a homogeneous group needs to be challenged while recognizing that each subgroup brings their own social, political, historical, and cultural context into the new setting.

Meanwhile, in communities where few Latinos have resided in the past, all four arenas of accessibility seem critically important. These communities are most likely in their infancy in creating alcohol-related services that are culturally appropriate and, thus, meet the needs of the growing Latino population. In designing social services, organizations must be cognizant that accessibility extends beyond having the services. Delgado's (2002) four arenas of accessibility can be a useful tool for organizations in these communities as they start designing alcohol-related services for the growing Latino population.

### Multicultural Training

Multicultural training is changing in the context of the twenty-first century. Paulino (1994) states that, "Increasing ethnic diversity in the United States carries with it important implications for the effective delivery of social services to people of color" (p. 53). Moreover, "Culturally competent substance abuse treatment service delivery refers to clinicians and agencies that demonstrate knowledge, values, and skills for working with individuals from a different cultural background" (Paz, 2002, p. 126). A complete overview of multicultural training towards the goal of culturally competent alcohol services is not the aim of this section. Rather there are issues that need to be raised regarding multicultural training in the context of what has been presented thus far.

Gloria and Peregoy (1996) present a model of cultural values and issues that need to be addressed when working with Latino alcohol and other drug users. Notwithstanding within group heterogeneity they discuss Latino shared cultural beliefs such as *influencia de la family*/family influence, *simpatía*/congenial, *personalismo*/personalism, *los papeles de género*/gender roles, and *espiritismo*/spiritualism. Several of these factors have previously been acknowledged in the literature. Paulino (2002) looking at human services for Dominicans discusses in detail the role of family and family dynamics in the United States. Delgado (1998) also recognizes the role of family in alcohol and other drug-related services. Paz (2002) also outlines several issues that are necessary for training culturally competent clinicians that work with the Latino population.

Elements that are important for training culturally competent providers to work with Latinos across the board have been widely discussed in the literature. However, the framework for training culturally competent practitioners needs to be revisited. There are important issues that arise in light of recent demographic shifts. One underlying assumption in culturally competent training is that we are training members of different cultural groups to work with another group. This type of training takes on a cross-cultural perspective. As a result of the growing diversity of Latinos already discussed, the model for multicultural training needs to also incorporate modules for intragroup training. There is a need to acknowledge that training that assumes shared Latino values, cultural beliefs, and other elements is not sufficient. There are differences among the Latino subgroups represented in the United States that require attention. This training needs to be targeted not only to providers that are non-Latino, but also to specific Latino subgroups, meaning that a Puerto Rican clinician might benefit from specific training around Guatemalan immigrants' cultural, historical, social, and political background. These types of training need to happen on a regular basis as efforts continue to enhance culturally appropriate alcohol-related services for a rapidly growing population.

## *CONCLUSION*

Alcohol-related problems remain a concern for the Latino population. Caetano and Clark (1998) state that in the past few years there has been an overall reduction in alcohol consumption in the United States. Latinos, however, are experiencing this reduction differently than their White counterparts. Caetano and Clark (1998) further note that for Whites there seems to be a switch from heavy to lighter drinking, with levels of abstention remaining relatively stable, while for Latinos rates of heavy drinking have remained stable over the years. Alcohol-related services remain a high priority for the Latino population.

In the past ten years, the Latino population has significantly increased. More poignant is not just the increase in relative size, but it's growing diversity. It is therefore of great interest for alcohol-related practitioners to remain in tune with these changes as they seek to enhance services. The main purpose of this brief overview of demographics has been to paint a portrait of the Latino population in the twenty-first century, while simultaneously outlining key implications for alcohol-related services. As we move forward in the twenty-first century, it is time to enhance existing cultural competency frameworks for working with Latinos as well as continue to build on the knowledge base by incorporating the population's growing complexity.

## REFERENCES

Caetano, R. & Clark, C.L. (1998). Trends in alcohol consumption patterns among Whites, Blacks, and Hispanics: 1984 and 1995. *Journal of Studies on Alcohol, 59,* pp. 659-667.

Cohn, D. (2002, July 31). Area Latino population among tops in growth. *The Washington Post.* Retrieved October 8, 2003, from *http://web.lexis-nexis*

De La Rosa, M.R. (2000). An analysis of Latino poverty and a plan of action. *Journal of Poverty, 4,* pp. 27-62.

Delgado, M. (1997). Hispanics/Latinos. In J. Philleo & Brisbane, F.L. (Eds.), *Cultural competence in substance abuse prevention* (pp. 33-50). Washington, DC: NASW Press.

Delgado, M. (1998). *Social services in Latino communities.* Binghamton, NY: The Haworth Press.

Delgado, M. (2002). Latinos and alcohol: Treatment considerations. *Alcoholism Treatment Quarterly, 20,* pp. 187-192.

Gloria, A.M. & Peregoy, J.J. (1996). Counseling Latino alcohol and other substance users/abusers. *Journal of Substance Abuse Treatment, 13,* pp. 119-126.

Guzmán, B. (2001). The Hispanic population: Census 2000 brief. U.S. Department of Commerce: Washington, DC.

Hobbs, F. & Stoops, N. (2002). U.S. Census Bureau, Census 2000 Special Reports Series CENSR-4, Demographic Trends in the 20th Century. U.S. Government Printing Office: Washington, DC.

Hollman, F. & Mulder, T. (2000, January 13). Census bureau projects doubling of nation's population by 2100. U.S. Department of Commerce: Washington, DC.

Kail, B., Zayas, L.H. & Malgady, R.G. (2000). Depression, acculturation, and motivations for alcohol use among young Colombian, Dominican, and Puerto Rican Men. *Hispanic Journal of Behavioral Sciences, 22,* 64-77.

Kilty, K.M. & Vidal de Haymes, M. (2000). Racism, nativism, and exclusion: Public policy, immigration, and the Latino experience in the United States. *Journal of Poverty, 4,* 1-25.

Kitchen, J. (2002). The Hispanic boom. *Hispanic, 15,* pp. 32-34.

Martínez-Brawley, E.E. & Zorita, P.M-B. (2001). Immigrants, refugees, and asylum seekers: The challenge of services in the southwest. *Journal of Ethnic & Cultural Diversity in Social Work, 10,* pp. 49-67.

Mayo-Quiñones, Y. & Helfgot, R.P.R. (2003). Immigrant Latino populations in the Untied States: Developing a cross-cultural perspective for social work education. *The Social Work Forum, 36,* pp. 35-57.

National Institute on Drug Abuse. (2003). Drug use among racial/ethnic minorities (NIH Publication No. 03-3888). Bethesda, MD: National Institute on Drug Abuse.

Neilsen, A.L. (2000). Examining drinking patterns and problems among Hispanic groups: Results from a national survey. *Journal of Studies on Alcohol, 61*, pp. 301-310.

Neilsen, A.L. (2001). Drinking in adulthood: Similarities and differences in effects of adult roles for Hispanic ethnic groups and Anglos. *Journal of Studies on Alcohol, 62*, pp. 745-749.

Paulino, A. (1994). Dominican in the United States: Implications for practice and policies in the human services. *Journal of Multicultural Social Work, 3*, pp. 53-65.

Paz, J. (2002). Culturally competent substance abuse treatment with Latinos. *Journal of Human Behavior in the Social Environment, 5*, 123-136.

Portes, A. & Rumbaut, R.G. (1996). *Immigrant America: A portrait.* Berkeley: University of California Press.

Proctor, B.D. & Delaker, J. (2002, September). Poverty in the United States: 2001. Current Population Reports, P60-219, U.S. Government Printing Office: Washington, DC.

Rodriguez-Andrew, S. (1998). Alcohol use and abuse among Latinos: Issues and examples of culturally competent services. In M. Delgado (Ed.), *Alcohol use/abuse among Latinos* (pp. 55-70). New York: Haworth Press.

Strug, D.L. & Mason, S.E. (2002). Social service needs of Hispanic immigrants: An exploratory study of the Washington Heights community. *Journal of Ethnic and Cultural Diversity in Social Work, 10*, pp. 69-88.

Suárez-Orozco, M.M. & Páez, M.M. (2002). Introduction: The research agenda. In M.M. Suárez-Orozco & M.M. Páez (Eds.), *Latinos remaking America* (pp.1-27). Berkeley, CA: University of California Press.

Suro, R. (2002, May 9). Counting the "other Hispanics": How many Colombians, Dominicans, Ecuadorians, Guatemalans, and Salvadorans are there in the United States. Pew Hispanic Center: Washington, DC.

Suro, R. & Passel, J.S. (2003, October). The rise of the second generation: Changing patterns in Hispanic population growth. Pew Hispanic Center: Washington, DC.

Therrien, M. & Ramirez, R.R. (2001). The Hispanic population in the United States: Population characteristics. Current Population Reports. U.S. Department of Commerce: Washington, DC.

U.S. Census Bureau (2003, March 21). Women edge men in high school diplomas, breaking a 13-year deadlock. U.S. Department of Commerce: Washington, DC.

Vega, W.A. (1990). Hispanic families in the 1980s: A decade of research. *Journal of Marriage and the Family, 52*, 1015-1024.

Vega, W.A., Gil, A.G. & Kolody, B. (2002). What do we know about Latino drug use? Methodological evaluation of state databases. *Hispanic Journal of Behavioral Sciences, 24*, pp. 395-408.

Wall, S. (2003, June 19). Latino population surges in U.S.: Growth is four times overall national rate. *San Bernandino County Sun.* Retrieved October 8, 2003, from *http://web.lexis-nexis.com*

Zhou, M. (2002). The changing face of America: Immigration, race/ethnicity, and social mobility. In P.G. Min (Ed.), *Mass migration to the United States* (pp. 65-98). Walnut Creek, CA: AltaMira Press.

# SECTION 2:
# PREVENTION AND TREATMENT

Chapter 3

# Seeking Care for Alcohol Problems: Patterns of Need and Treatment Among Mexican-Origin Adults in Central California

William A. Vega, PhD
William M. Sribney, PhD

**SUMMARY.** Alcohol dependence is a serious problem in the Mexican-origin population of the United States. While the magnitude of these problems is well documented, the use of services and their relative effectiveness in accessing and treating alcohol dependence have been inade-

William A. Vega is Professor of Psychiatry, Robert Wood Johnson Medical School, and Director, Division of Research, Behavioral Research and Training Institute–University Behavioral HealthCare, 151 Centennial Ave., Piscataway, NJ 08854 (E-mail: vegawa@umdnj.edu).

William M. Sribney is a biostatistician at University Behavioral HealthCare.

[Haworth co-indexing entry note]: "Seeking Care for Alcohol Problems: Patterns of Need and Treatment Among Mexican-Origin Adults in Central California." Vega, William A., and William M. Sribney. Co-published simultaneously in *Alcoholism Treatment Quarterly* (The Haworth Press, Inc.) Vol. 23, No. 2/3, 2005, pp. 29-51; and: *Latinos and Alcohol Use/Abuse Revisited: Advances and Challenges for Prevention and Treatment Programs* (ed: Melvin Delgado) The Haworth Press, Inc., 2005, pp. 29-51. Single or multiple copies of this article are available for a fee from The Haworth Document Delivery Service [1-800-HAWORTH, 9:00 a.m. - 5:00 p.m. (EST). E-mail address: docdelivery@haworthpress.com].

doi:10.1300/J020v23n02_03

quately studied. This paper describes patterns of care for alcohol disorders by examining the distribution of alcohol dependence and utilization rates, and identifying population characteristics that influence perceived need and receipt of treatment. *[Article copies available for a fee from The Haworth Document Delivery Service: 1-800-HAWORTH. E-mail address: <docdelivery@haworthpress.com> Website: <http://www.HaworthPress.com> © 2005 by The Haworth Press, Inc. All rights reserved.]*

**KEYWORDS.** Latinos, Mexican Americans, alcohol dependence, alcohol services, alcohol treatment

## *INTRODUCTION*

Considerable attention has been devoted to mental health services for Latinos with mental illnesses, yet little attention has focused on treatment for alcohol problems. As a result there is only limited information about the characteristics of individuals with alcohol problems, their beliefs and opinions about providers, usual sources of care, or estimates about the proportion of met and unmet need for treatment. What information is available from national survey data indicates Latinos were more likely than European Americans to receive less care than needed or delayed care, 10.7% vs 22.7%, and were less satisfied with substance abuse treatment they received (Wells, Klap, Koike, and Sherbourne, 2001). The need for more research on patterns of care for alcohol problems among Latinos has been noted in the research literature, especially descriptive research on client characteristics, pathways to care, access barriers and treatment preferences (Caetano, 1993). This study examines treatment patterns using a community epidemiologic sample of adults residing in Central California that were of Mexican origin and about evenly distributed between immigrants and U.S. born (Vega, Kolody, Aguilar-Gaxiola, Alderete, Catalano, and Caraveo-Anduaga, 1998).

Past research has shown variability in alcohol problems across Latino nationality groups, with Mexican-origin people having the highest rates of alcohol abuse or dependence and a mortality rate for alcohol-related cirrhosis (13.3 per 100,000) that is far higher than for African Americans (8.3) or European Americans (5.2) (Dawson, 1998; NIAAA, 1991). Although a large proportion of Puerto Rican and Cuban males use alcohol they are less prone toward frequent heavy drinking than those of Mexican origin (Caetano, 2001). Mexican-origin men have much higher alcoholism rates than women; however, alcohol dependence rates for women of Mexican-origin increase between the first and second generations in the U.S. (Caetano, 2001; Vega, Kolody, Aguilar-Gaxiola, Alderete, and Caraveo-Anduaga; Catalano, 1998). Acculturation is important because the longer immigrants reside in the United States the greater the likelihood of alcohol dependence, yet Latinos who immigrated as children have higher rates than other immigrants–and are similar to U.S.-born Latinos (Turner and Gil, 2002; Vega, Sribney, Aguilar-Gaxiola, and Kolody, 2004).

There are additional burdens that accompany alcohol dependence such as higher rates of spousal abuse, co-occurring psychiatric disorders, illicit drug abuse or dependence, tobacco dependence, and high arrest rates for alcohol-related offenses, especially DUI violations (Vega, Sribney, Achara-Abrahams, and Vega, 2001; 2003; Regier, 1990; Chambless, Cherney, Caputo, and Rheinstein, 1987). Indeed, among Mexican immigrants fully one-half of all arrests are attributable to drunk driving, as are one-third of all arrests for the U.S. born (Vega, 2001). These encounters with the criminal justice system often lead to detention and paradoxically a primary source of care–court-ordered therapy. Alcohol dependence also has negative effects on health status, disability, employment status, and income (Seale, Williams, and Amodei, 1992). In sum, excessive alcohol consumption is a serious, endemic problem with multiplier effects in the Latino population. Preventing alcohol abuse and effectively treating those who are alcohol dependent can lower the burden of disease and is an important public health goal.

While it is a normal start point to evaluate the gap between Latinos who are alcohol dependent and how many receive treatment in various settings, an even more utilitarian question is why some perceive a need for assistance of some type while others do not, and why do some help-seekers actually receive treatment while others fail to do so. These are key questions in Latino behavioral health services research which are repeatedly asked, yet few empirical studies have actually attempted to answer them (Vega, Kolody, and Aguilar-Gaxiola, 2001; Pescasolido, McLeod, and Alegria, 2000; Portes, Kyle, and Eaton, 1992; Alegria et al., 1991). Help-seeking involves a combination of individual, family, social network, community, and health-care system characteristics that interact in a complex fashion over time and are difficult to measure, analyze, and interpret (Anderson, 1995). Help-seeking models are optimally useful when explanations follow a logical sequence of events. It is admittedly difficult to do this with cross-sectional data because these events can unfold over many years in an idiosyncratic, unsystematic sequence. This has posed a longstanding limitation for contemporary research.

Bearing these limitations in mind, we present descriptions of the various types of providers and services received by Mexican-origin adults with alcohol abuse or dependence, their perceptions about the effectiveness and acceptability of receiving care, and nested models that explore which perceptions and other factors influence perceived need and receipt of treatment. We have followed the procedures used by Mojtabai, Olson, and Mechanic (2002) in their recent article on perceived need using the National Comorbidity data set. They created nested multivariate models to predict both perceived need and receipt of treatment. Perceived need as formulated by these researchers and in this study is based on indirect self-report and self-directed behaviors, as described in the methods section. Perceived need is a subjective construct and differs from objective need because the latter is based on external criteria such as medical protocols. Perceived need as we define it herein would be expected to vary across subgroups and individuals, in contrast, objectively defined need would be invariant.

## METHODS

Study participants were part of an epidemiologic sample of $N = 3,012$ persons, all of Mexican origin, from the Fresno, California, Mexican American Prevalence and Services Survey (Vega et al., 1998). The sample was selected under a fully probabilistic, stratified, multistage cluster design. Subjects were weighted by the inverse of their selection probability, and weights were adjusted to conform the sample to the Fresno County census age-sex distribution for Mexican-origin adults. After the study was explained, a written informed consent was obtained. Face-to-face field interviewing was conducted in 1996. The response rate was 90% among screened eligible households. A full description of the design of this study and data-collection methods can be found in Vega et al. (1998).

The Composite International Diagnostic Interview (Wittchen et al., 1991), a fully structured clinical inventory using DSM-III-R diagnostic criteria, was the diagnostic protocol used in this study and was administered by trained lay interviewers. DSM-III-R diagnoses were determined for the following disorders: alcohol abuse or dependence, nonalcohol drug abuse or dependence, major depressive episode, manic episode, dysthymia, panic disorder, agoraphobia, social phobia, simple phobia, and antisocial personality disorder. "Nonsubstance-use mental disorder" comprises one or more of the last seven diagnoses. Subjects who responded with symptoms of substance-use disorders (either alcohol or drugs or both) were asked whether they sought or received treatment for their substance use; treatment responses were not specific to the type of substance used (i.e., treatment could be for either alcohol or drugs or both).

Tables 1 and 2 give prevalence estimates calculated as the weighted subsample sum for those with the listed characteristic or diagnosis divided by the total weighted subsample sum. All standard error estimates were adjusted for the sampling design through a first-order Taylor series approximation, and significance probabilities in Table 2 for the pairwise differences of the utilization rate estimates were calculated using Wald tests (Cochran, 1977; StataCorp, 2001). All estimates from the models of Tables 3 and 4 account for the weighted, stratified, and clustered sampling design and were computed using the svy commands of Stata 7.0 (StataCorp, 2001).

Table 3 gives responses adjusted for sex, age (18-24, 25-34, 35-44, or 45-59 years), marital status (married, divorced/separated/widowed, or never married), urban versus rural or town, education (0-6 years versus 7+), and family income (< $12,000 versus $12,000+). Responses were modeled using logistic regression (questions 3-7), ordered logistic regression (questions 1 and 8), multinomial logistic regression (question 9), and linear regression (question 2) with independent variables consisting of the four categories shown in Table 3 (alcohol abuse/dependence or not for immigrants and U.S. born) and the adjustment covariates (sex and age were retained in all models regardless of significance; other covariates were only retained if $p < 0.05$). Table 3 gives predicted probabilities from these models expressed as percentages for the reference category of male, age 25-34, married, urban, 7+ years of education, and $12,000+ family income. Significance tests for nativity and diagnosis differences were based on Wald tests derived from model estimates.

## RESULTS

Table 1 shows the study sample characteristics. About 60% were immigrants and 40% were U.S. born, and the U.S.-born sample was relatively younger. Twice as many immigrants (14%) had family incomes of less than $6,000 as U.S. born (7%), and over twice as many U.S. born (47%) as immigrants (21%) had incomes of $18,000 or more. Self-reported language preference showed that 52% of immigrants and only 4% of U.S.-born adults prefer to speak only Spanish. Table 1 also shows the lifetime prevalence of DSM-III-R alcohol abuse or dependence with or without other co-occurring diagnoses. Among U.S.-born males, the

TABLE 1. Sample characteristics[a] (*N* = 3,012) and lifetime prevalence of DSM-III-R alcohol abuse or dependence with or without drug abuse or dependence and with or without nonsubstance-use mental disorders[b] by nativity and sex.

| | Immigrants | | | U.S. born | | |
|---|---|---|---|---|---|---|
| | Female | Male | Total | Female | Male | Total |
| Observed sample | 912 | 922 | 1834 | 604 | 574 | 1178 |
| Weighted sample percentage | 44.8 | 55.2 | 60.1 | 49.4 | 50.6 | 39.9 |
| Age (y) | | | | | | |
| 18-24 | 21.6 | 21.1 | 21.3 | 27.9 | 35.1 | 31.5 |
| 25-34 | 40.2 | 38.6 | 39.3 | 27.1 | 28.1 | 27.6 |
| 35-44 | 22.0 | 23.0 | 22.6 | 24.9 | 21.8 | 23.3 |
| 45-59 | 16.1 | 17.3 | 16.7 | 20.2 | 15.0 | 17.6 |
| Family income ($) | | | | | | |
| < 6,000 | 15.8 | 13.3 | 14.4 | 7.0 | 7.3 | 7.2 |
| 6,000-11,999 | 42.3 | 32.1 | 36.7 | 25.8 | 19.6 | 22.6 |
| 12,000-17,999 | 27.1 | 28.3 | 27.8 | 24.6 | 22.8 | 23.7 |
| 18,000-35,999 | 10.4 | 17.2 | 14.2 | 25.1 | 24.2 | 24.7 |
| ≥ 36,000 | 4.3 | 9.1 | 7.0 | 17.6 | 26.0 | 21.9 |
| Language preference[c] | | | | | | |
| Spanish all of the time | 59.7 | 46.3 | 52.3 | 2.9 | 5.2 | 4.1 |
| Spanish most of the time | 15.6 | 18.0 | 16.9 | 6.3 | 5.0 | 5.7 |
| Spanish and English equally | 21.1 | 28.1 | 24.9 | 24.1 | 22.8 | 23.4 |
| English most of the time | 3.2 | 6.2 | 4.9 | 33.8 | 44.9 | 39.4 |
| English all of the time | 0.4 | 1.5 | 1.0 | 32.9 | 22.1 | 27.5 |
| Alcohol abuse/dependence without any other disorders | 0.0 | 9.1 | 5.0 | 4.0 | 12.3 | 8.2 |
| Alcohol abuse/dependence with drug abuse/dependence[d] | 0.2 | 2.0 | 1.2 | 1.1 | 6.0 | 3.6 |
| Alcohol abuse/dependence with nonsubstance-use mental disorder[b,e] | 0.7 | 3.5 | 2.2 | 4.8 | 5.5 | 5.1 |
| Alcohol abuse/dependence with drug abuse/dependence and nonsubstance-use mental disorder[b] | 0.5 | 1.2 | 0.9 | 3.7 | 6.7 | 5.2 |
| Total alcohol abuse/dependence[f] | 1.5 | 15.8 | 9.4 | 13.7 | 30.4 | 22.1 |

[a] All data except sample counts are reported as percentages.
[b] Nonsubstance-use mental disorders include DSM-III-R mood, anxiety, and antisocial personality disorders.
[c] Native Mexican languages included in "Spanish" categorization.
[d] Without any nonsubstance-use mental disorder.
[e] Without drug abuse/dependence.
[f] Total alcohol abuse/dependence with or without other disorders.

TABLE 2. Lifetime utilization rates[a] of treatment providers and services for persons with DSM-III-R lifetime alcohol abuse or dependence with or without co-occuring nonsubstance-use mental disorders[b] by nativity.

| | Treatment of substance-use disorder[c] | | | | Treatment of nonsubstance-use mental disorder | |
|---|---|---|---|---|---|---|
| | Alcohol abuse/dependence without nonsubstance-use mental disorder | | Alcohol abuse/dependence with nonsubstance-use mental disorder | | Alcohol abuse/dependence with nonsubstance-use mental disorder | |
| Type of provider/service | Immigrants[d] | U.S. born[e] | Immigrants[d] | U.S. born[e] | Immigrants | U.S. born |
| Mental health specialist (including psychiatrist)[f] | 1 | 7* | 2 | 17** | 13 | 41** |
| Medical doctor (other than psychiatrist) | 6 | 28** | 2 | 22*** | 17 | 34 |
| Hospitalized for substance use | 5 | 12 | 4 | 10 | 5 | 12 |
| Medicated for substance use | 1 | 11* | 0 | 6 | 16 | 33* |
| Any medical provider/service (any of above) | 11 | 34** | 7 | 35*** | 35 | 63* |
| Other professional[g] | 8 | 15 | 3 | 18 | 33 | 34 |
| Folk/natural healer, spiritualist, psychic, astrologist, santero(a), and/or sobabor(a) | 0 | 0 | 1 | 1 | 15 | 18 |
| Herbal remedies, prayers, blessed water, baths, cleansings, sorcery, and/or exorcism | 5 | 6 | 13 | 10 | 35 | 43 |
| Self-help group, not court ordered | 6 | 14* | 17 | 22 | - | - |
| Self-help group, court ordered | 33 | 14* | 21 | 26 | - | - |
| Any provider/service | 50 | 54 | 44 | 60 | 56 | 84* |

[a] Rates reported as percentages.
[b] Nonsubstance-use mental disorders include DSM-III-R mood, anxiety, and antisocial personality disorders.
[c] Treatment of substance-use disorder includes treatment for alcohol use, drug use, or both.
[d] Among immigrants with alcohol abuse/dependence, all differences in rates of treatment of substance abuse/dependence between those with nonsubstance-use mental disorder and those without nonsubstance-use mental disorder were not significant.
[e] Among U.S. born with alcohol abuse/dependence, all differences in rates of treatment of substance abuse/dependence between those with nonsubstance-use mental disorder and those without nonsubstance-use mental disorder were not significant.
[f] Includes psychiatrists, psychologists, social workers, psychiatric nurses, and mental health workers.
[g] Includes priests, ministers, rabbis, counselors, nurses, chiropractors, and homeopaths.
* $p < 0.05$, ** $p < 0.01$, *** $p < 0.001$, for difference of U.S. born and immigrant.

TABLE 3. Attitudes[a] toward mental health treatment for persons with and without[b] DSM-III-R lifetime alcohol abuse or dependence by nativity.

| Question | Alcohol abuse/dependence | | No alcohol abuse/dependence[b] | |
|---|---|---|---|---|
| | Immigrants | U.S. born | Immigrants | U.S. born |
| 1. How comfortable would you feel talking about personal problems with a professional? | | | | |
| Very | 42.5 | 28.0 | 43.4 | 32.6 |
| Somewhat | 37.5 | 39.8 | 37.2 | 39.8 |
| Not very | 12.9 | 19.6 | 12.6 | 17.3 |
| Not at all | 7.0 | 12.6 | 6.8 | 10.4 |
| | c | c | d | d |
| 2. Suppose that 10 people are receiving treatment from a professional for serious emotional or mental health problems. Of these 10 people, how many do you think are helped? | 6.7[c] | 4.9[c,e] | 7.0[d] | 5.7[d,e] |
| 3. If you needed help for an emotional or mental health problem, would you | | | | |
| a. Know where to obtain help or treatment? | 40.6[c] | 66.6[c] | 42.7[d] | 63.1[d] |
| b. Have transportation to get there? | 91.7 | 94.0[e] | 94.3[d] | 97.2[d,e] |
| c. Have someone to go with? | 83.2 | 89.9 | 87.7[d] | 91.5[d] |
| d. Not want to get help because of having to take time off from work? | 26.3 | 29.0 | 22.3 | 27.3 |
| e. Not want to get help because of any other reasons? | 3.3[c] | 12.8[c] | 4.1[d] | 8.7[d] |
| 4. Do you feel that most family physicians can be a great help with an emotional or mental health problem? | 76.6 | 68.1 | 76.7[d] | 65.4[d] |
| 5. If you sought help, do you think a mental health professional would understand the kinds of problems that you might have? | 90.8 | 82.5[e] | 94.7[d] | 91.4[d,e] |
| 6. If you had an emotional or mental health problem, would you find talking to a priest, minister, or rabbi as useful as talking to a mental health specialist? | 35.5 | 41.9 | 34.1[d] | 45.5[d] |
| 7. Would you avoid treatment of emotional or mental health problems because your friends might find out? | 3.6 | 8.9 | 5.0 | 6.5 |
| 8. How would you rate the quality of mental health care available to you? | | | | |
| Excellent | 9.1 | 8.1 | 17.4 | 14.8 |
| Good | 39.2 | 37.1 | 49.0 | 47.1 |
| Fair | 41.3 | 43.2 | 28.4 | 31.9 |
| Poor | 10.3 | 11.5 | 5.2 | 6.2 |
| | f | e | f | e |
| 9. If you went for treatment, would you prefer speaking in | | | | |
| Spanish | 54.9 | 1.6 | 60.7 | 2.3 |
| English | 9.7 | 70.4 | 3.9 | 66.2 |
| Both | 35.4 | 28.0 | 35.4 | 31.5 |
| | c | c | d | d |

[a] Answers shown as percentages, adjusted for sex, age, marital status, urban vs. rural or town, education, and family income, for the reference category of male, age 25-34, married, urban, 7+ years of education, and $12,000+ family income (see text). Percentages for questions 3-7 are percentages of "yes" responses.
[b] Persons with nonalcohol drug abuse/dependence are excluded from the "no alcohol abuse/dependence" reference category.
[c] Difference between immigrants with alcohol abuse/dependence and U.S. born with alcohol abuse/dependence significant ($p < 0.05$).
[d] Difference between immigrants without alcohol abuse/dependence and U.S. born without alcohol abuse/dependence significant ($p < 0.05$).
[e] Difference between U.S. born with alcohol abuse/dependence and U.S. born without alcohol abuse/dependence significant ($p < 0.05$).
[f] Difference between immigrants with alcohol abuse/dependence and immigrants without alcohol abuse/dependence significant ($p < 0.05$).

TABLE 4. Odds ratios [95% confidence intervals] from logistic regressions (modeled separately by nativity) of a model of perceived need for persons with DSM-III-R lifetime alcohol abuse or dependence and a model for treatment for those persons with perceived need.

| | Perceived need model for persons with alcohol abuse/dependence (Sought or received services or self-reported limitation vs. neither) | | Treatment model for persons with perceived need (Sought or received medical treatment[a] vs. sought or received other services or self-reported limitation only) | |
|---|---|---|---|---|
| | Immigrants | U.S. born | Immigrants | U.S. born |
| Number of persons | 167 | 240 | 84 | 156 |
| **Sociodemographic variables** | | | | |
| Sex | | | | |
| Female | 2.3 [0.3, 17] | 2.6 [0.9, 7.5] | 1.1 [0.1, 22] | 0.8 [0.3, 2.1] |
| Male | 1 | 1 | 1 | 1 |
| Age (y) | | | | |
| 18-24 | 1.1 [0.2, 7.0] | 0.4 [0.1, 1.3] | 1.1 [0.1, 12] | 0.8 [0.2, 3.4] |
| 25-34 | 1 | 1 | 1 | 1 |
| 35-44 | 1.2 [0.4, 3.6] | 1.1 [0.3, 3.4] | 1.4 [0.3, 7.6] | 0.2 [0.1, 0.8]* |
| 45-59 | 0.6 [0.1, 4.2] | 0.8 [0.2, 2.8] | 0.4 [0.0, 5.0] | 2.0 [0.4, 9.8] |
| Years in U.S. | | | | |
| < 13 | 1.1 [0.3, 3.6] | NA | 1.3 [0.1, 21] | NA |
| ≥13 | 1 | | 1 | |
| Language preference for treatment | | | | |
| Spanish | 8.8 [2.3, 33]** | | 1.5 [0.1, 32] | |
| English or both | 1 | | 1 | |
| Spanish or both | | 2.8 [1.2, 6.6]* | | 1.3 [0.5, 3.1] |
| English | | 1 | | 1 |
| Education (y) | | | | |
| 0-6 | 0.7 [0.2, 2.0] | | c | |
| 7+ | 1 | | | |
| 0-11 | | 2.5 [1.0, 6.2]* | | 0.4 [0.2, 1.3] |
| 12+ | | 1 | | 1 |
| Family income ($) | | | | |
| <12,000 | 1.5 [0.6, 3.6] | | 1.0 [0.2, 5.5] | |
| 12,000+ | 1 | | 1 | |
| <18,000 | | 0.7 [0.3, 1.7] | | 1.2 [0.4, 3.7] |
| 18,000+ | | 1 | | 1 |

37

TABLE 4 (continued)

| | Perceived need model for persons with alcohol abuse/dependence | | Treatment model for persons with perceived need | |
| | (Sought or received services or self-reported limitation vs. neither) | | (Sought or received medical treatment[a] vs. sought or received other services or self-reported limitation only) | |
| | Immigrants | U.S. born | Immigrants | U.S. born |
|---|---|---|---|---|
| Place of residence | | | | |
| Town or rural | 2.0 [0.6, 6.6] | 1.1 [0.5, 2.3] | 1.8 [0.3, 13] | 0.1 [0.1, 0.4]*** |
| Urban | 1 | 1 | 1 | 1 |
| Health insurance | | | | |
| Public assistance | 0.3 [0.1, 1.4] | 2.1 [0.6, 7.3] | 2.9 [0.2, 36] | 1.5 [0.4, 5.3] |
| Other | 0.6 [0.2, 1.9] | 1.7 [0.6, 5.0] | 5.5 [1.1, 28]* | 0.9 [0.2, 3.5] |
| No insurance/don't know | 1 | 1 | 1 | 1 |
| **Severity/comorbidity** | | | | |
| Number of alcohol-use disorder symptoms | | | | |
| ≥ 5 | 16.4 [5.1, 52.6]*** | 6.1 [2.4, 16]*** | 1.2 [0.1, 11] | 0.6 [0.2, 1.5] |
| < 5 | 1 | 1 | 1 | 1 |
| Comorbid drug abuse/dependence | | | | |
| Yes | 2.4 [0.5, 11] | 15.1 [4.5, 51]*** | 6.2 [0.6, 67] | 1.0 [0.4, 2.4] |
| No | 1 | 1 | 1 | 1 |
| Comorbid nonsubstance-use mental disorder[b] | | | | |
| Yes | 0.4 [0.1, 1.2] | 0.6 [0.3, 1.4] | 0.5 [0.1, 2.2] | 1.4 [0.6, 3.8] |
| No | 1 | 1 | 1 | 1 |
| **Physical health** | | | | |
| Severe physical health problem lifetime | | | | |
| Yes | 0.9 [0.3, 2.8] | 1.4 [0.6, 3.7] | 6.8 [1.6, 29]** | 3.7 [1.4, 9.8]** |
| No | 1 | 1 | 1 | 1 |

**Attitudes**

| | | | |
|---|---|---|---|
| How comfortable talking about personal problems with a professional? | | | |
| Very or somewhat | 1 | 1 | 1 | 1 |
| Not very or not at all | 2.9 [0.9, 9.6] | 2.4 [1.0, 5.6]* | 0.5 [0.1, 2.6] | 4.1 [1.2, 14]* |
| Number of people who you think are helped out of 10 receiving treatment from a professional for mental health problems | | | | |
| ≥ 6 | 1 | 1 | 1 | 1 |
| < 6 | 0.1 [0.0, 0.3]*** | 0.6 [0.3, 1.5] | 1.1 [0.1, 11] | 1.4 [0.6, 3.5] |

**Social support/experiences**

| | | | |
|---|---|---|---|
| Have someone to share innermost thoughts and feelings or problems? | | | | |
| Yes | 1 | 1 | 1 | 1 |
| No | 0.3 [0.1, 0.9]* | 1.0 [0.4, 2.4] | 1.3 [0.2, 6.9] | 3.3 [1.0, 11]* |
| Have family, relatives, or friends to drive you somewhere, loan you $50, or comfort you? | | | | |
| Almost all or some of the time | 1 | 1 | 1 | 1 |
| Rarely or little of the time | 0.5 [0.2, 1.6] | 1.1 [0.5, 2.7] | 1.1 [0.2, 5.9] | 2.9 [0.9, 9.5] |
| Have you been discriminated against? | | | | |
| Yes | 0.1 [0.0, 0.5]** | 1.2 [0.5, 3.1] | c | 0.8 [0.3, 2.0] |
| No | 1 | 1 | 1 | 1 |

[a] Medical treatment of substance-use disorder includes treatment for alcohol use, drug use, or both, and includes services sought or received from mental health specialists or medical doctors, hospitalization for substance use, and medication for substance use.
[b] Mental disorders include DSM-III-R mood, anxiety, and antisocial personality disorders.
[c] Variable not included in model because variable was nearly collinear with other (nonsignificant) variables. Variable was not significant when added to a model that included only significant variables.
NA, not applicable.
* $p < 0.05$, ** $p < 0.01$, *** $p < 0.001$.

prevalence of alcohol abuse or dependence is 30% and among immigrant males 16%. The majority of U.S.-born males with alcohol abuse or dependence have another DSM-III-R diagnosis, whereas the majority of male immigrants with alcohol abuse or dependence have only this disorder. The prevalence of alcohol abuse or dependence is very low among female immigrants (< 2%), but the prevalence among U.S.-born females (14%) is almost the same as that for immigrant males. Over two-thirds of U.S.-born females with alcohol abuse or dependence have another DSM-III-R diagnosis.

Table 2 shows lifetime utilization rates of treatment providers and services for persons with alcohol abuse or dependence by nativity. The first four columns of data give rates for treatment sought or received for substance use. During the survey, persons with symptoms of alcohol abuse or dependence were asked whether they sought or received treatment for alcohol use; persons with symptoms of alcohol abuse or dependence and nonalcohol drug abuse or dependence were asked whether they sought or received treatment for their alcohol or drug use without specificity to the substance used. Hence, those responses shown in the first four columns of data in Table 2 include treatment of alcohol use, drug use, and both alcohol and drug use. Rates are given for persons with alcohol abuse/dependence and a nonsubstance-use mental disorder and for those without a nonsubstance use mental disorder. The last two columns of Table 2 give rates for the treatment of any nonsubstance-use mental disorder for those with alcohol abuse/dependence and a nonsubstance-use mental disorder. Immigrants and U.S. born show very different patterns of treatment for substance use. Immigrants are far less likely to use medical providers or services (first five rows of data in Table 2). However, immigrants with alcohol abuse/dependence and no nonsubstance-use mental disorder are more likely to have the experience of a court-ordered self-help group. Utilization of providers and services for substance-use treatment were very similar among those with and without a nonsubstance-use mental disorder, and no significant differences were found. The rate of utilization of medical providers and services for a nonsubstance-use mental disorder differ between immigrants (35%) and U.S. born (63%) with both alcohol abuse/dependence and a nonsubstance-use mental disorder, but the relative difference here is much smaller than the corresponding rates in the same groups for medical treatment of substance use (7% for immigrants and 35% for U.S. born).

Table 3 gives responses for questions reflecting attitudes toward mental health treatment for persons with and without alcohol abuse/dependence. Since responses to these questions were significantly related to sociodemographic factors, these factors were controlled for using logistic regression and other modeling procedures (see Methods). Hence, Table 3 shows responses adjusted for sex, age, marital status, urban versus rural or town, education, and family income.

Immigrants are more likely than U.S. born to give positive responses about potential interactions with professionals concerning mental health problems (questions 1 and 5 of Table 3), and are more likely to anticipate positive outcomes from treatment (questions 2 and 4). Immigrants, however, rate talking to a priest, minister, or rabbi concerning mental health problems less useful than talking to a mental health professional than do U.S. born (question 6). Differences between those with and without alcohol abuse/dependence for these six questions were only significant for questions 2 and 5 and only for U.S. born. U.S. born with alcohol abuse/dependence were the least optimistic about the proportion of persons helped by mental health treatment (question 2) and least likely to think that mental health professionals would understand the kinds of problems that they might have (question 5), although the level of positive responses to this last question were still quite high. Less than ten percent of persons said that they would avoid treatment of mental health problems because their friends might find out (question 7), and there were no significant differences among the subgroups shown in Table 3. Persons with alcohol abuse/dependence gave significantly lower ratings of the quality of mental health care available to them (question 8) than did those without alcohol abuse/dependence; however, immigrants and U.S. born gave remarkably similar ratings. Language preference for treatment shown in Table 3 follows general language preferences given in Table 1: few of the U.S. born desire treatment in Spanish and few of the immigrants desire treatment in English.

Table 4 gives two models concerning perceived treatment need for persons with alcohol abuse/dependence (first two columns of data) and seeking or receipt of medical services for those with a perceived need (last two columns), fit with separate logistic regressions for immigrants and U.S. born. The dependent variable for the perceived need model is positive if either (1) the person sought or received treatment from any provider or service (i.e., the category of the last row of Table 2), or (2) the person reported limitation(s) caused by alcohol use (possibly in conjunction with drug use or a nonsubstance mental disorder). This self-reported limitation was indicated by any positive response to the question *Do problems with your use of alcohol [and drugs and mental health] seriously limit any major life activity such as managing money, communicating, doing everyday household chores, or going outside the home alone?* or a response of either "a lot," "some," or "a lit-tle," to the question *How much do problems with your use of alcohol [and drugs and mental health] limit you in doing things that most peo-ple your age are able to do?* ("drugs" and "mental health" were in-cluded in the question if the respondent had earlier expressed symptoms of nonalcohol drug abuse/dependence or nonsubstance-use mental dis-order in addition to symptoms of alcohol abuse/dependence).

Of the 17 independent variables of the perceived need model for im-migrants, five were significant. In the model for U.S. born, five out of 16 terms were significant. Immigrants with alcohol abuse/dependence who preferred treatment in Spanish were far more likely (odds ratio 8.8 for comparison with English or both Spanish and English) to have a per-ceived need for treatment than those who preferred treatment in English or both languages. U.S. born who preferred treatment in Spanish or both Spanish and English were similarly more likely to have a perceived need than those preferring treatment in English (odds ratio 2.8). Educa-tion has significance for U.S. born, but not for immigrants. For both im-migrants and U.S. born, severity of alcohol dependence as indicated by the number of symptoms for the disorder was highly predictive of need. Comorbid drug abuse/dependence had a large, highly significant odds ra-tio (15.1) for U.S. born, but the corresponding odds ratio for immigrants was not significant, although elevated (2.4).

Odds ratios for expressing comfort about personal problems with a professional (question 1 from Table 3) are similar in immigrants (2.9) and U.S. born (2.4), although only the one for U.S. born achieved sig-nificance. In contrast, optimistic responses to proportion of persons helped by mental health treatment (question 2 from Table 3) have a highly significant association with lower perceived need in immigrants (odds ratio 0.1); this term also had an odds ratio of less than one in the U.S. born, but did not reach significance. These two questions were chosen for the model because they had the greatest significance of any of the items in Table 3.

In immigrants, greater levels of social support (*having someone to share innermost thoughts and feelings or problems* and *having family, relatives, or friends to drive you somewhere, loan you $50, or comfort you*) are associated with lower levels of perceived need, although only the first of these two questions reached significance. In the U.S. born, no association for these two questions was seen. "Yes" responses to the question *Have you been discriminated against?* have a highly signifi-cant association with lower perceived need in immigrants (odds ratio 0.1), but there is no such association in the U.S. born.

The second model in Table 4 is nested within the first. This treatment model has as dependent variable whether persons with a perceived need sought or received medical services for substance-use disorder (the "any medical provider/service" category of Table 2). Of the 16 independent variables in the model for U.S. born, five were significant. Of the 15 independent variables in the model for immigrants, only two were significant. Two variables, education and perceived discrimination, that were included in the model for perceived need had to be omitted from the treatment model for immigrants because they were nearly collinear with other variables in the model (all of which were nonsignificant). When education and perceived discrimination were added to a model consisting of only significant variables, they were nonsignificant.

The age group 35-44 was associated with a lower rate medical treatment in the U.S. born; however, its statistical significance was only marginal, and it is likely just a chance occurrence of the sampling. Place of residence was highly significant for the U.S. born, with persons residing in rural or town areas less likely to seek or receive medical treatment than urban dwellers (odds ratio of 0.1). For immigrants, persons residing in rural or town areas were more likely to seek or receive medical treatment (odds ratio of 1.8), although this association did not reach significance. Among immigrants, having health insurance was associated with being more likely to seek or receive medical treatment, but insurance in the U.S. born appeared to have no association with medical treatment rates. Interestingly, severity of alcohol dependence seemed not to affect who sought or received medical treatment. Having a severe physical health problem, however, had a highly significant association with greater rates of medical treatment in both immigrants and U.S. born. This association is largely due to the fact that persons with severe physical health problems are more likely to seek or receive services from doctors other than psychiatrists (odds ratio of 12.5, $p = 0.01$, for immigrants; odds ratio of 3.4, $p = 0.01$, for U.S. born).

The attitude question concerning comfort talking about personal problems with a professional was again significant in the U.S. born, with those expressing a greater level of comfort more likely to seek or receive medical treatment. For the U.S. born, having someone to share innermost thoughts and feelings also made a person more likely to seek or receive medical treatment. Attitudes and social support, however, seemed to have no effect on medical treatment rates for immigrants.

## DISCUSSION

This study has examined patterns of care among Mexican-origin people who have reported alcohol abuse or dependence in their lifetimes. We hasten to add that our "lifetime" approach to both prevalence and treatment histories is unorthodox. Most studies report only one-year rates because they are more accurate than lifetime recall. While it is obvious why recall of recent utilization is more accurate, we used a lifetime approach because we believe it to be much more informative for depicting patterns in a population that is disproportionately immigrant with very low utilization rates. The findings suggest that many Mexican-origin people with serious alcohol problems do not receive adequate treatment, and this includes both immigrants and Mexican Americans (U.S. born). The findings of this study reiterate the evident distinctions between Latino immigrants and U.S.-born Latinos regardless of nationality. Immigrants tend to retain the language and culture of origin tenaciously, especially if they immigrated as adults. U.S.-born Latinos such as Mexican Americans emulate substance use behavior of the U.S. population. These generalizations seem pertinent to alcohol consumption patterns as reflected in prevalence rates of alcohol dependence disorders and co-occurring disorders.

Mexican Americans have consistently higher dependence rates than immigrants and thus have a higher need for services. However, immigrants *with* alcohol abuse or dependence disorders have lower utilization rates for all types of services, except folk remedies and court-ordered self-help groups, compared to Mexican Americans with alcohol disorders. Court-ordered self-help groups are the primary source of care for immigrants with serious alcohol problems. Alcohol dependent immigrants *who also have co-occurring mood, anxiety, or antisocial personality disorders* have a similar low likelihood (7%) of seeking or receiving medical treatment for substance-use as those without a co-occurring disorder, even though their rates of medical treatment for their nonsubstance-use mental disorders (35%) are relatively much closer to that of U.S. born.

Overall, our findings underscore that Mexican immigrants are marginal to the health care system compared to Mexican Americans. Their linguistic and cultural insularity seemingly provides protective effects for them against substance disorders to a certain extent though this is less true of alcohol use than it is for drugs, but this protection is not fully transferable to the next generation. The higher rates for alcohol dependence among Mexican American women, as contrasted with minimal alcoholism among immigrant women, illustrate this point. Despite having higher treatment rates than immigrants, the higher prevalence of alcohol dependence among Mexican Americans indicates that they too are underserved, especially in rural and small town areas where options to court-ordered treatment are in short supply.

## Access Barriers, Prevention, and Recovery

The high prevalence of untreated alcohol dependent individuals imposes a burden of disease on the Latino community that is staggering. Our results suggest that the severity of alcohol symptoms are often very advanced before individuals perceive a need for treatment, and this is especially true for immigrants. One of the major obstacles to more effective treatment of alcohol and related problems for Latinos has been and continues to be their lack of access to care. Though it is a story often repeated, it is undeniable that the compounding of low socioeconomic status and labor concentration in sectors unlikely to provide employer-sponsored health insurance, lessens the likelihood that emergent and chronic health conditions such as alcohol addiction will be effectively treated (Falcon, Aguirre-Molina, and Molina, 2001). Studies of mental health care utilization point to insurance availability as a critical factor distinguishing which Latinos receive treatment (Vega, Kolody, and Aguilar-Gaxiola, 2001).

However, factors other than insurance availability may also influence the access to care. Our results show (counterintuitively) that immigrants are more likely than Mexican Americans with alcohol abuse or dependence to believe treatment from a professional provider would be beneficial, but Mexican Americans are more likely to know where to obtain that treatment yet have more personal reasons, including stigma, for not seeking it. Therefore, a complex picture emerges about acceptability of treatment that is likely rooted in personal experience with the treatment system and information gained from social network interaction. Most notable is the preference of immigrants for Spanish language treatment that is difficult to access.

The Latino community doubtless needs community campaigns to reduce the stigma of alcohol treatment and other co-occurring disorders, and promote early identification of alcoholism and timely alcohol treatment. Community educational programs that "normalize" treatment for behavioral health conditions have shown promise of being useful for mental health problems in other settings and cultures (Paykel, Hart, and Priest, 1998; Jorm, 2000). However, these strategies are weakened without access to care, availability of Spanish-speaking treatment staff for immigrants, and culturally competent treatment practices to reduce treatment avoidance due to past negative interactions with the treatment system. Greater pessimism about the worth of alcohol treatment may arise because a high percentage of alcohol-dependent Mexican Americans have co-occurring disorders involving illicit drugs and have been "turned-off" by previous experiences with substance-abuse treatment providers. Mexican Americans with alcohol abuse or dependence were roughly 3 times more likely to receive medical treatment if they reported feeling comfortable about talking with professionals about their personal problems.

The research literature is consistent in reporting that Latino and non-Latino patients receiving care for alcoholism have similar clinical features regarding severity of disease progression, drinking practices, and dysfunction (Arciniega, Arroyo, Miller, and Tonigan, 1996). However, the research evidence is mixed and fragmentary about what treatments work best for Latinos with alcohol dependence, and the weight of research suggests that both type of provider and modality of intervention are important. There is a general impression in the literature, buttressed by empirical confirmation, that standard Alcoholics Anonymous group meetings do not work as well with Latinos as they do with European Americans, yet empirical evidence is lacking regarding what other modalities of group or cognitive behavioral therapy are more effective with Latinos (Arroyo, Miller, and Tonigan, 2003; Hall, 2001). One reason for this is because studies are needed with samples of adequate statistical power to permit identification of Latino client characteristics that predict better outcomes when matched with specific modalities of treatment. Although it has been reported that acculturation does not appear to predict treatment outcome, it is difficult with small samples to avoid confounding of acculturation with demographic factors especially when clients are relatively homogeneous on factors such as socioeconomic status, nativity/nationality, and gender.

## Cultural Competence and Alcohol Treatment for Latinos

There is very little research on the role, value, or most appropriate implementation of culturally competent practices, including overcoming linguistic barriers and translation issues, family integration into therapy, and improving acceptability and treatment satisfaction with services (Hall, 2001; Gil, Wagner, and Tubman, 2003). The identification of cultural competence factors that are most effective for increasing access to care or that improve treatment outcomes have not been systematically studied. This literature will undoubtedly grow exponentially in the coming years as standards in culturally competent care are formulated and disseminated by public and private bodies, implemented by health care agencies, and enforced by accrediting bodies. Albeit limited, there is evidence that utilization, quality, and effectiveness of substance abuse services are improved through the use of culturally competent treatment practices, but much more needs to be learned about best practices in clinical care, treatment planning, medication adherence, and how to provide linguistic/culturally competent care (Campbell and Alexander, 2002).

In alcohol treatment of Latinos, a logical start point is to discuss the special characteristics of the Latino population as these potentially affect the willingness to seek treatment, selection of treatment settings, successfully accessing treatment and receiving appropriate care, forming a workable therapeutic relationship, staying in treatment long enough to benefit from it, and effectively responding to relapse. However, while remaining mindful of ethnic group social and cultural factors, it is equally important to keep in mind that treatment always focuses on the individual and her/his needs and characteristics. While individuals may reflect aspects of group experience and cultural orientations, by no means are they consistent in the way they do so. As a way of formulating a strategy for addressing alcohol treatment with Latinos, we have borrowed liberally and extended the treatment framework recommended by Gil, Wagner, and Tubman (2003). We believe culturally competent treatment practices should cover the interplay of "surface" psychosocial indicators, such as socioeconomic status, acculturation status (Hispanic/Latino vs. American, cultural orientation, ethnic identity), nativity, language preferences, cultural beliefs and practices (low vs. high distress threshold, time orientation, interpersonal relationships), acculturation stress (actual and/or perceived discrimination, individual acculturative stress, family acculturative stress), developmental status (life course stage, developmental trajectory in the U.S.).

However, these indicators are cardinal points, they do not constitute a treatment strategy. Since therapeutic models are usually developed for non-Latino populations based on their cultural expectations and tolerance levels, even basic issues such as accessibility of location, bilingual staffing, and respect and consideration of cultural beliefs and expectations should be carefully considered. Then, a second step is required to address "core" issues using the surface indicators as "probes" to formulate a culturally appropriate treatment plan. This strategy "connects the dots" by systematically linking cultural characteristics to the individual; for example, examine immigration history, acculturation level and acculturation stress, ethnic identity, familial elements, and traditional cultural values in their unique individual expression, including assessing unique needs and strengths of U.S. born and immigrant Hispanic/Latinos. Next consider, differential levels of acculturation within the family; "amenability-to-treatment" issues when using "off-the-shelf" interventions and how these correspond to unique cultural factors expressed by the client; cultural orientation and relational style (e.g., individualistic vs. family), reciprocity expectations, relational style (e.g., warm/empathetic, business-like/rational); level of life stress, history of trauma, acculturation stress, discrimination, and modes of cultural interpretation and coping; cultural expectations about treatment; problem orientation of the client; and focus on concrete present-oriented factors.

## Establishing Models for Best Practices in Primary Care

As is the case with mental health treatment, primary care is a customary setting for accessing and treating the Latino population regardless of socioeconomic status because it is the most frequently used provider (Seale, Williams, and Admodei, 1992). Given the relatively high percentage of Latinos, especially males, who have some degree of serious drinking problems, and our findings suggest that severe physical health problems increase the likelihood of receiving alcohol treatment, it is especially useful to implement routine screening in primary care for alcoholism. Efficient screening instruments are now available for use in primary care settings to protect physician time. Primary care physicians are a trusted medical care provider and a major referral source for specialized treatment among Latinos, and research studies have reported success in screening and treating clients with alcoholism (Burge, Amodei, Elkin, Catala, Andrews, Lane, and Seale, 1997).

Additional interventions may be required in successfully identifying and treating co-occurring medical problems, tobacco dependence, and psychiatric disorders that are frequently found in alcohol abusing populations (Vega, Sribney, and Achara-Abrahams, 2003). Failure to address multiple disorders with a coordinated treatment plan can frustrate recovery from alcohol dependence and perpetuate functional impairments and self-destructive behavior (Merikangas et al., 1998). The major issues include recognizing that co-occurring disorders are present through accurate diagnosis, coordinating appropriate services so that the treatment planning is effective, avoiding medication complications, and educating family members about what to expect over the course of treatment. This will increase family members' cooperation, and decrease potential misunderstanding and role strains.

## *CONCLUSION*

This study has profiled the lifetime use of different types of behavioral health services by Mexican immigrants and Mexican Americans with alcohol dependence, including those with additional co-occurring behavioral health problems such as illicit drug dependence, mood, and anxiety disorders. The prevalence of alcohol disorders is much higher among Mexican Americans than it is among immigrants. While Mexican Americans receive significantly more medical and other therapeutic services than immigrants, neither group received adequate treatment. Indeed, the primary source of care for immigrants with alcohol problems is attendance at court-ordered (DUI) groups. The research on alcohol treatment with Latinos is consistent in reporting Latinos are less receptive to AA groups than European Americans; however, there is inadequate empirical evidence about what treatment modalities are preferred or most effective with Latinos.

Populations with high concentrations of immigrants have special requirements because they have low access to care, are culturally distinctive, and most immigrants need or prefer Spanish language services. This underscores the problem of how to access them, especially in the subgroup where alcoholism is most concentrated, among males, yet they are the least likely to use voluntary therapeutic services. The treatment literature offers an important insight, effective screening and treatment can be implemented in primary care clinics that are perhaps the most promising setting for regular access to Latinos and ostensibly invoke less stigma. It is also encouraging that immigrants are not more dubious than are Mexican Americans in believing professional therapy is a useful form of care. The problems remain of overcoming access barriers such as lack of insurance, knowing how and where to access care, and finding culturally/linguistically competent therapists. However, these problems are not as serious in primary care because it is the most universal and preferred provider for Latinos. In sum, a complex picture emerges of differences between immigrants and U.S. born in perceiving a need for care and in receiving treatment for alcohol dependence. The current body of research on utilization and treatment is too limited to form any firm conclusions about "best practices" for alcohol dependent Latinos. The rapid population growth and the implicit acceleration of unmet need for treatment among Latinos will hopefully serve as a wake-up call to address unmet need among federal research agencies and public or private treatment providers.

## REFERENCES

Alegria, M. et al. (1991) Patterns of mental health utilization among island Puerto Rican poor. Amer J Pub Heal 81:875-879.

Anderson, R.M. (1995) Revising the behavioral model and access to medical care. J Heal Soc Behav 36:1-10.

Arciniega, L.T., Arroyo, J.A., Miller, W.R., Tonigan, J.S. (1996) Alcohol, drug use and consequences among Hispanics seeking treatment for alcohol related problems. J Stud Alcohol 57:613-8.

Arroyo, J.A., Miller, W.R., Tonigan, J.S. (2003) The influence of Hispanic ethnicity on long-term outcome in three alcohol treatment modalities. J Stud Alcohol 64:98-104.

Arroyo, J.A., Westerberg, V.S., Tonigan, J.S. (1998) Comparison of treatment utilization and outcome for Hispanics and non-Hispanic whites. J Stud Alcohol 59:286-91.

Burge, S.K., Amodei, N., Elkin, B., Catala, S., Andrew, S.R., Lane, P.A., Seale, J.P. (1997) An evaluation of two primary care interventions for alcohol abuse among Mexican American patients. Addiction 12:1705-16.

Caetano, R., Galvan, F.H. (2001) Alcohol use and alcohol related problems among Latinos in the United States. In M. Aguirre-Molina, C.W. Molina, and R.E. Zambrana (ed.), Health Issues in the Latino Community, San Francisco, CA: Jossey-Bass; pp.381-412.

Caetano, R., Schafer, J. (1996) DSM-IV alcohol dependence in a treatment sample of White, Black, and Mexican American men. Alcohol Clin Exp Res 20:384-90.

Caetano, R. (1993) Priorities for alcohol treatment research among U.S. Hispanics. J Psychoactive Drugs 25:53-60.

Campbell, C.I., Alexander, J.A. (2002) Culturally competent treatment practices and ancillary service use in outpatient substance abuse treatment. J Sub Abuse Treatment 22:109-119.

Chambless, D., Cherney, J., Caputo, G., Rheinstein, B. Anxiety disorders and alcoholism: A study of inpatient alcoholics. J Anxiety Disorders 1:29-40.

Cochran, W.G. (1977) Sampling Techniques, 3rd ed. New York: John Wiley & Sons.

Dawson, D.A. (1998) Beyond Black, White, and Hispanic: Race, ethnic origin and drinking patterns in the United States. J Subst Abuse 10:321-339.

Gil, A.G., Wagner, E., Tubman, J. (2003) Culturally sensitive substance abuse intervention for Hispanic and African American adolescents: Empirical example from the "ATTAIN" project. Unpublished manuscript. Florida International University.

Falcon, A., Aguirre-Molina, M., Molina, C.W. (2001) Latino health policy: Beyond demographic determinism. In M. Aguirre-Molina, C.W. Molina, and R.E. Zambrana (ed.), Health Issues in the Latino Community, San Francisco, CA: Jossey-Bass; pp.3-22.

Hall, G.C.N. (2001) Psychotherapy research with ethnic minorities: Empirical, ethnical, and conceptual issues. J Consult Clin Psycho 69:502-510.

Jorm, A.F. (2000) Mental health literacy: Public knowledge and beliefs about mental disorders. Br J Psychiatry 177:396-401.

Merkangas, K.R., Mehta, R.L., Molnar, B.E. et al. (1998) Comorbidity of substance use disorders with mood and anxiety disorders: Results of the International Consortium in Psychiatric Epidemiology. Addict Behav 23:893-907.

Mojtabai, R., Olfson, M., Mechanic, D. (2002) Perceived need and help-seeking in adults with mood, anxiety, or substance use disorders. Arch Gen Psychiatry 59:77-84.

NIAAA (1991) Liver cirrhosis mortality in the United States: 1970-86. Bethesda, MD: Surveillance Report 52.

Paykel, E.S., Hart, D., Priest, R.G. (1998) Changes in public attitudes to depression during the Defeat Depression Campaign. Br J Psychiatry 173:519-522.

Pescasolido, B.A., Wright, E.R., Alegria, M., Vera, M. (1998) Social networks and patterns of use among the poor with mental health problems in Puerto Rico. Medical Care 36:1057-1072.

Portes, A., Kyle, D., Eaton, W.W. (1992) Mental illness and help-seeking behavior among Mariel Cuban and Haitian refugees in South Florida. J Heal Soc Behav 33:283-298.

Regier, D.A., Farmer, M.E., Rae, D.S. et al. (1990) Comorbidity of mental disorders with alcohol and other drug use. JAMA 264:2511-2518.

Seale, J.P., Williams, J.F., Amodei, N. (1992) Alcoholism prevalence and utilization of medical services by Mexican Americans. J Fam Pract 35:169-74.

StataCorp (2001) Stata Statistical Software Release 7.0. College Station, TX: Stata Corporation.

Turner, R.J., Gil, A.G. (2002) Psychiatric and substance use disorders in South Florida. Arch Gen Psychiatry 59:43-50.

Vega, W.A., Sribney, W.M., Aguilar-Gaxiola, S., Kolody, B. (2004) 12-month prevalence of DSM-III-R psychiatric disorders among Mexican Americans: Nativity, social assimilation, and age determinants. J Nerv Ment Dis (in press).

Vega, W.A., Sribney, W.M., Achara-Abrahams, I. (2003) Co-occurring alcohol, drug, and other psychiatric disorders among Mexican-origin people in the United States. AJPH 93:1057-1064.

Vega, W.A., Kolody, B., Aguilar-Gaxiola, S. (2001) Help seeking for mental health problems among Mexican immigrants and Mexican Americans. J Immigrant Health 3:133-140.

Vega, W.A., Kolody, B., Aguilar-Gaxiola, S., Alderete, E., Catalano, R., Carveo-Anduaga, J. (1998) Lifetime prevalence of DSM-III-R psychiatric disorders among urban and rural Mexican Americans in California. Arch Gen Psychiatry 55:771-778.

Vega, W.A. (2001) A profile of crime, violence, and drug use among Mexican immigrants. Perspect Crime Justice (National Institute of Justice) 4:51-68.

Wells, K., Klap, R., Koike, A., Sherbourne, C. (2001) Ethnic disparities in unmet need for alcoholism, drug abuse, and mental health care. Am J Psychiatry 158:2027-2037.

Wittchen, H.U., Robins, L.N., Cottler, L.B., Sartorius, N., Burke, J.D., Regier, D. (1991) Cross-cultural feasibility, reliability, and sources of variance of the Composite Diagnostic Interview (CIDI). Br J Psychiatry 195:645-653.

Chapter 4

# Alcohol Use Among Dominican-Americans: An Exploration

Annecy Baez, CSW, PhD

**SUMMARY.** Research on alcohol use among Mexicans, Puerto Ricans and Cubans has benefited from the general and positive research trend towards disaggregating data that was historically collected on Hispanics as a whole (Black & Markides, 1994; Canino, 1994; Canino et al., 1992; Kail et al., 2000; Lee et al., 1997; Nielsen, 2000; Randolph et al., 1998; Wells et al., 2001). But as the representation of other Hispanic groups in the United States escalates rapidly, alcohol research agendas have been slow to incorporate these groups on a larger scale, with Dominicans being a prime example. This chapter explores the Dominican presence in the United States, Dominican culture, and the limited research specific to Dominicans and alcohol use. *[Article copies available for a fee from The Haworth Document Delivery Service: 1-800-HAWORTH. E-mail address: <docdelivery@haworthpress.com> Website: <http://www.HaworthPress.com> © 2005 by The Haworth Press, Inc. All rights reserved.]*

**KEYWORDS.** Latinos, Dominicans, alcohol

---

Annecy Baez is Associate Professor of Social Work at New York University School of Social Work, 1 Washington Square North, New York, NY 10003 (E-mail: annecy.baez@nyu.edu).

[Haworth co-indexing entry note]: "Alcohol Use Among Dominican-Americans: An Exploration." Baez, Annecy. Co-published simultaneously in *Alcoholism Treatment Quarterly* (The Haworth Press, Inc.) Vol. 23, No. 2/3, 2005, pp. 53-65; and: *Latinos and Alcohol Use/Abuse Revisited: Advances and Challenges for Prevention and Treatment Programs* (ed: Melvin Delgado) The Haworth Press, Inc., 2005, pp. 53-65. Single or multiple copies of this article are available for a fee from The Haworth Document Delivery Service [1-800-HAWORTH, 9:00 a.m. - 5:00 p.m. (EST). E-mail address: docdelivery@haworthpress.com].

Available online at http://www.haworthpress.com/web/ATQ
© 2005 by The Haworth Press, Inc. All rights reserved.
doi:10.1300/J020v23n02_04

## INTRODUCTION

### The Dominican Presence in the United States

The Dominican Republic, with its 8.1 million inhabitants, is the product of diverse racial influences that begins with the Taino Indians, whose influence remains today in the names of foods, towns and the Taino name for the island, still commonly used, *Quisqueya*, which means "the mother of all lands."

The African influence in Dominican culture has been felt in agriculture, religion and spiritual practices (Baez & Hernandez, 2001). The Spanish influence is prominent in the national language and in many customs. It is less well known that Dominican cultural diversity reaches still further, to include Italians, Germans, Sephardic Jews from Curacao, Jewish refugees from Europe, Puerto Ricans, Cubans, West Indians, Chinese, Japanese and Lebanese. All of these diverse ethnic groups have intermingled to create modern Dominican culture (Alcantara et al., 1995; Chapman, 1997; Torres-Saillant & Hernandez, 1998).

Dominicans are clearly prominent among the newer Hispanic immigrant populations in the United States. The fastest rate of growth in recent years is not in the historically largest Hispanic groups (Mexicans, Puerto Ricans, and Cubans), but among Dominicans (now the 4th largest group), Salvadorans, Colombians and other peoples from Central and South America (Logan, 2001). The U.S. Census 2000 tally of 764,495 Dominicans is nonetheless considered significantly undercounted. Castro and Boswell (2002) estimate the actual number of Dominicans at 1,014,879, while Logan (2001) estimates the number to be 1,121,257. The Dominican Diaspora is a relatively recent event, with 71.1% of all native Dominicans in the U.S. immigrating from 1980 to 2000, the highest among Hispanic groups in this country. Dominicans in the U.S. are also a markedly youthful population, with 22.9% of the Dominican population in the U.S. ten years of age or younger, 44.2% under twenty, and 59% under thirty (Castro & Boswell, 2002).

The Dominican population in the U.S. is highly concentrated, with 85% residing in the vicinity of just six major metropolitan areas: New York/Northern New Jersey (67%), Miami/Fort Lauderdale (7.7%), Boston/Worcester (4.1%), Los Angeles/Riverside (3.5%), Philadelphia/Wilmington (1.7%) and Houston/Galveston (1.2%). New York City is the epicenter of the Dominican presence in the U.S., and Dominicans are the city's largest and fastest growing immigrant population.

Educational attainment figures for Dominicans in this country reflect an improving, but still woefully inadequate situation, with just 9.6% achieving a Bachelor's degree. In the U.S. as a whole, by comparison, 24.8% of the population has a BA degree. Reflecting the strong Dominican values around youth and education, U.S. born Dominicans are faring better, with a BA attainment rate of 21.7% (Castro & Boswell, 2002). Educational achievement is inhibited by the fact that in many of the U.S. urban areas where Dominicans reside, they often receive an inferior education in public primary and secondary schools plagued by shortages of teachers, high teacher turnover, lack of adequate supplies, overcrowded classes and poor building maintenance (Anyon, 1997). It is not uncommon for Dominican students in these areas to have taken five or six years to complete high school (Lopez, 2002). Economically, Dominicans stand out for their very low income. Many earn below $8,000 (Logan, 2001) and 45.7% live below the poverty line (Hernandez & Torres Saillant, 1997). On average, Dominican women earn approximately 25% less than their male counterparts (Castro & Boswell, 2002). Duany (1994) points to the frequent struggles of New York City based Dominicans, even by the standards of recent immigrants, for fair wages and decent housing.

Dominicans thus share with their Hispanic immigrant counterparts conditions that put them and their children at greater psychosocial risk for negative social, health, and developmental outcomes: poor education, employment at lower paying jobs, and high rates of poverty (Zayas, 1992).

## The Expanding Scope of Research on Hispanic Ethnic Groups and Drinking Behavior

As is the case in many other areas of research, Nielsen and Ford (2001) noted that "there has been, until recently, very little research that has examined alcohol use by Hispanics, despite the population's growth and youth." They point out, as do others (Gilbert and Cervantes, 1986; Dusenbury, 1994; Caetano et al., 1998), the potential for significant differences in drinking patterns across Hispanic ethnic group that cannot be successfully analyzed until there are more studies that disaggregate by Hispanic ethnicity. The need for such studies is clear. In 1999, the most common substance abuse problem among Hispanics was alcohol (SAMSHA, 2003), accounting for 36% of all Hispanic substance abuse problems. Caetano and Clark (1998) found that prevalence of alcohol problems among Hispanics increased from 1984 to 1995, while there was no change among African Americans or whites. Although factors other than alcoholism contribute to the higher death rates from cirrhosis and liver disease among Hispanics in comparison to non-Hispanics, alcoholism is prominent on the list (Sorlie, 1993).

Recent studies on alcohol use by Hispanics have thus understandably focused on the largest Hispanic groups, Mexicans, Cubans, and Puerto Ricans (Aquirre-Molina & Caetano, 1994; Canino et al., 1992; Black & Markides, 1994; Canino, 1994; Lee et al., 1997; Randolph et al., 1998; Kail et al., 2000; Nielsen, 2000; Wells et al., 2001). But changing population trends in the U.S. now call for a significant broadening of the scope of Hispanic groups studied, with Dominicans being a prime example. One dominant theme that has emerged in research on drinking patterns among all ethnic groups in the U.S. is the contributing influence of stressors related to social adjustment to life in the U.S. (Caetano et al., 1998). Al-Issa (1997) highlights acculturative stress, socio-economic stress, and minority/racism-based stress as being prominent in this regard. Other highly significant factors include norms and attitudes (Oostveen et al., 1996; Alva & Jones, 1994), situational norms (Greenfield & Room, 1997; Caetano & Clark, 1998), and social influence (Dusenbury, 1994). Given this emerging understanding, there will follow an overview of Dominican American culture with the intent of searching for points of convergence and differentiation from generalized attributes of Hispanic culture, as well as for emerging understanding about norms, attitudes, social influence, and stress factors that may help to illuminate the relationship between Dominicans and drinking behavior. This overview is offered as an orientation for clinicians and researchers who may be less familiar with Dominican culture, and is offered with a full understanding that culture and ethnicity in reality has a dynamic, diverse and multidimensional nature that such overviews cannot do full justice to (Betancourt & Lopez, 1993; Phinney, 1996).

### Cultural Characteristics of Dominicans in the United States

Dominicans generally share with other Hispanic groups adherence to important norms and customs which serve as guides for conduct: the centrality of family life as an area of obligation and interdependence, adherence to traditional gender roles, the value of showing respect, and the importance of both Christian and complementary (i.e., Espiritismo & Santeria) spiritual beliefs (Baez & Hernandez, 2001). Regarding the last point, complementary and alternative medical and spiritual practices, Allen et al. (2000) found that nearly half of Dominican patients presenting at a New York City emergency room had used indigenous medicine, usually in the form of medicinal plants and herbal teas, for their presenting complaints. Observance of life cycle markers and appropriate rituals are a similarly central feature: birthday celebrations, religious rituals, wedding anniversaries, even Sunday picnic traditions, are all treated with reverence and call for almost obligatory attendance (Falicov, 1999). In a study of Dominicans, social relations, and depression, LaRoche (1999) found that family life was the context in which Dominicans obtained most of their supportive social interactions.

Certain nuances of Dominican family life merit further explanation because they differ dramatically from non-Hispanic American family life, and to a lesser extent from family life in other Hispanic cultures. It is important to bear in mind that Dominican family boundaries very often include non-blood relatives, most significantly the *hijo/hija de crianza* (a "child of upbringing" or informally adopted child) and the *compadre/comadre* (godparent or co-parent). These members are active participants in family life and are generally subject to the same expectations and privileges as blood relatives, so much so that a sexual liaison between a *compadre* and his godchild is virtually unheard of, and is considered tantamount to incest. Three marriage forms are generally viewed as acceptable: civil, religious, and free union. While some free unions last a lifetime, their potential disadvantage become apparent in situations where men leave the household due to affairs or economic pressures, leaving the women with limitations in terms of legal recourse to support themselves and their children (Hernandez, 1997).

Among the other features that to some degree distinguish Dominicans from other Hispanics are Dominican determination to preserve their culture and identity, and the high frequency of travel between the United States and the Dominican Republic (Iltis, 2001). This is convergent with Grasmauck and Pessar's (1991) observation that Dominican rates of U.S. naturalization are historically low. Duany (1994) and Georges (1989) also highlight the *transnational* nature of the Dominican community; the ambivalent attachment that Dominicans have with the U.S. and the Dominican Republic, as well as their frequent travel between the countries, and their commitment to sending money (an estimated 500 million dollars a year) and material goods back home (Sontag & Dugger, 1998).

Cosgrove (1992) points to another noteworthy aspect of the relatedness many Dominicans have with the two countries: the phenomenon of *remigration*, wherein significant numbers of Dominicans emigrate to the U.S., then after a period of years, they remigrate from the U.S. to the

Dominican Republic. Some of these *retornos* or "returners" may even repeat this pattern more than once. Cosgrove believes that Dominicans are perhaps "the most outstanding example" of this practice, and as a Dominican American woman, this writer's experience is that this practice occurs much more frequently with Dominicans than with other Hispanic groups.

Among the effects of this transnational Dominican style may be a slowing of acculturation and assimilation. Substantial numbers of Dominicans live in the U.S. for many years and learn just a handful of English words during that time. Between the frequent travel, the abundance of money transfer companies and phone parlors in Hispanic neighborhoods, modems, fax machines, discount phone cards and long distance plans, the effect is such that families and cultural values remain intact (Georges, 1989; Baez, in press). This encapsulation of Dominican identity and cultural values, while strong, is not airtight, and tensions related to bicultural exposure sometimes make themselves apparent with Dominicans as they do with other Hispanic groups. This can be a good thing, an enriching experience that gives persons and families a wider set of adaptive resources, or it can be a source of difficulty and frustration as contradictory cultural views collide (Falicov, 1999). When children enter adolescence, for example, Dominican parents, like other Hispanic parents who often speak little English and have little understanding of American culture, may manifest overprotectiveness as they struggle to understand their children's interest in hip-hop fashion, numerous piercings for jewelry, and rap music.

### Dominican Men and Alcohol Use

In Dominican culture, the man is viewed as the head of the household. This places substantial pressures on a Dominican man to meet the needs of his family despite the limited economic opportunities, high cost of living, and sometimes intermittent employment that often confront him in this country. Given the centrality of family life for Dominicans, it is not commonly frowned upon as much for a man to have children from different relationships, but a man's failure to maintain those children is viewed as dishonorable. Thus, when a Dominican man is unable to provide fully for his family, leaving the family often becomes a preferable alternative. These pressures also places Dominican men at increased risk for depression and alcoholism (Kail et al., 2000). This finding can be seen as consistent with data from national surveys on drinking, which revealed that single Hispanic men were less likely to be current drinkers than those who were married (Caetano & Clark, 1998). While infidelity by married Dominican men is anecdotally believed to be a common problem, others point with pride to the increasing respect given to the *hombre serio* (Gordon, 1978) the serious or self-respecting Dominican man who devotes himself to hard work, family life and clean living.

As discussed earlier, poverty among Dominicans in the U.S. is high, educational attainment low, and the vast majority of Dominicans are found in just a few urban areas, all factors that are known to increase vulnerability to drug and alcohol use (SAMHSA, 1999). Yet surprisingly, a number of studies of Dominican adults have found the prevalence of alcohol use problems to be lower among Dominican adults than among other Hispanic adult groups.

In one of the earliest known American studies specifically on Dominicans and alcohol use, Gordon (1978) conducted an observational study of drinking behaviors of Dominican immigrants residing in Newton, Massachusetts. Situational norms regarding drinking in that community favored weekend consumption, in part because of weekday fatigue due to long hours worked. Wives were noted as a powerful social influence that seemed to successfully discourage frequent or heavy drinking in husbands in many cases. Contrary to the hypothesis that Dominican immigrants would manifest increased reliance on alcohol due to acculturative stress, Gordon found low rates of reliance on alcohol in the Newton Dominican community. Gordon attributed the lower rates to limits in time for socializing due to extended work schedules, limits in economic resources, and both religious and familial prohibitions against drinking in excess. More recently, a study conducted by Drohan et al. (1997) interviewed 210 Hispanics in a primary care setting using the Alcohol Use Disorders Identification Test, the CAGE questionnaire, and the Composite International Diagnostic Interview to determine past or present occurrences of alcohol abuse or dependence. They found the lifetime prevalence of these disorders among Dominicans to be 22%, while the prevalence for Central Americans was 41%, and for Puerto Ricans 47%. Zayas et al. (1998) interviewed 288 Puerto Rican, Dominican and Colombian men regarding depression and alcohol use. Dominicans were found to be at least risk among these participant groups for alcohol-related problems.

While encouraging, these studies are too few and too small in sample representation to allow for a conclusion that Dominicans are at low risk, or that they experience a low prevalence of alcohol-related problems, in comparison to other Hispanic groups. It is also possible that problem use of alcohol among Dominicans is low in comparison to other Hispanic groups, but still high in relation to non-Hispanic Americans. Alternatively, problem use of alcohol among Dominicans may be low in comparison to both Hispanic and non-Hispanic Americans, which could lead to studies of the protective factors that are contributing to this phenomenon. One possibility would be that the transnational nature of the Dominican Diaspora, the rapid rate of new arrivals from the Republic, combined with their settlement in just a few close-knit communities, may be converging to create an acculturative resistance that is advantageous in relation to problem use of alcohol among Dominican adults.

### Dominican Women and Alcohol Use

For many Dominican women in the United States, the world of work is often an exception to traditional gender roles; Dominican women enter the U.S. workforce in substantial numbers (Cosgrove, 1992) but often suffer under the strain of working full time while also being primarily responsible for child rearing, domestic chores, maintaining relations with extended family, and much more. An extraordinary 49% of New York City's Dominican households are headed by women (Hernandez & Torres Saillant, 1997; Ojito, 1997). In the author's clinical experience, women may leave relationships because of partner infidelity, inability of partners to provide economically, family violence, and sometimes to pursue new relationships that present themselves because of the fact that women have more socializing opportunities away from home.

Only about a third of alcohol abusing or alcohol dependent persons in the U.S. are women (Gordis, 1999). Caetano and Clark (1997), reporting on results from a national alcohol survey, indicated that the percentage of Hispanic women who abstain from alcohol rose from 47% in 1984 to 57% in 1995. Frequent heavy drinking among Hispanic women also increased in that same time period, from 2% to 3%. A study of Mexican women (Gilbert, 1987) found that reports of abstention from alcohol were greater among Mexican women who have immigrated to the U.S.; reports of moderate or heavy drinking were greater among younger, American-born women. This is convergent with Caetano's (1994) finding that U.S.-born Hispanic women are more likely to drink alcohol than Hispanic women that are immigrants. There is to date no substantive data on alcohol use by Dominican women. However, given the extraordinarily close relationship that many Dominicans maintain with their homeland (Georges, 1989; Baez, in press) and the steady stream of new immigrant arrivals to the U.S., it would not be surprising if use of alcohol in general, and problem use in particular, were found to be low.

## Dominican Adolescents and Alcohol Use

Numerous studies of inner-city youth indicate that exposure to traumatic life events and neighborhood disadvantage significantly predicts antisocial behavior and drug use among youth (D'Imperio et al., 2000; Dubow et al., 1997). This is a reality that appears to be intuitively understood by Dominican parents. In a 1998 *New York Times* article, educators and government officials in the Dominican Republic estimated that as many as 10,000 students from the United States are enrolled in Dominican schools, sent there by parents fearful of the dangers of urban street life in the U.S. In one school highlighted in the article, one in every five students was an American-born Dominican (Rohther, 1998). The country's recent ex-President, Leonel Fernandez Reyna, is also an example of the Dominican American transnational educational experience, having come to New York City with his immigrant mother, a seamstress and nurse's aide, at age eight.

The emerging data on Dominican youth and alcohol use paints a picture that is different from that of Dominican adults. Epstein et al. (2001) investigated alcohol use among Dominican and Puerto Rican sixth and seventh graders (849 at baseline, 678 at one year follow-up) and found Dominican adolescents generally engaged in comparatively higher rates of use. A study by Bettes et al. (1990) on over 2000 Black, Anglo, Dominican and Puerto Rican seventh graders reported that alcohol use was higher among the Dominican adolescents than the Puerto Rican adolescents, and higher among boys compared with girls.

Dusenbury et al. (1994) studied over 3,000 sixth and seventh graders in New York City whose ethnicity was Puerto Rican, Dominican, Colombian, Ecuadorian and other Hispanic. Dominican students, especially Dominican boys, had higher rates of drinking prevalence than the other groups. Boys in general tended to have higher alcohol use rates than girls. Dominican boys in particular had 3.22 times the odds of being a current drinker. The strongest predictor of drinking behavior measured in this study, far above predictors such as gender, academic performance, and parental attitudes towards drinking, was social influence. Having a few friends who drink increased the likelihood of a Dominican student exhibiting current drinking 7.84 times; having some to all friends who drink increased the odds 11.16 times.

## Conclusions

Findings on the most studied Dominican sub-population, adolescents in school, reveal an at risk population for whom culturally congruent prevention interventions need to be improved. Keeping in mind that 44% of Dominicans in the United States are under twenty years of age, and that high school dropout rates are high, research studies must also be extended into high school populations, and even more importantly, beyond school-based sampling.

The general trend in the extremely scarce research literature on Dominicans and alcohol use is that self-reported problem use among men appears to be low (although sample sizes have been small), the problem use of alcohol by Dominican women is statistically unknown, and alcohol use by adolescents in schools is an emerging problem.

A great deal about patterns of drinking behavior among Dominicans in this country remains unexplored and merits investigation. Very little is known about rates of abstention, consumption patterns, alcohol-related norms and attitudes, rates of frequent heavy drinking, and alcohol-related trends among Dominican women. While general indications are that prevalence of alcohol-related problems is low among Hispanic women, Dominican women lead high stress lives, with 49% the heads of their households, and those who are not heads of household laboring mightily to balance economic, familial and other demands.

Explorations of alcohol use among Dominicans would also benefit from expansion of the exploratory spectrum beyond the confines of self-reported use. Alcohol use is highly correlated with deaths from liver disease, homicides, home injuries, car accidents, family violence and child abuse (AMERSA, 2000). Research from these areas may shed considerable light on the extent to which alcohol use is a problem among Dominicans in this country.

## REFERENCES

Aguirre-Molina, M., & Caetano, R. (1994). Alcohol use and alcohol related issues. In C. W. Molina, and Aguirre-Molina, M. (Ed.), *Latino Health in U.S.: A Growing Challenge* (pp. 393-424). Washington, D.C.: American Public Health Association.

Alcantara, A., Aquino, J., Lantigua, J. A., Rodriguez, D., & Soto, A. (1995). *From Quisqueya: In search of new horizons: Dominican cultural heritage resource guide*. New York: Queens Borough Public Library.

Al-Issa, I. (1997). Ethnicity, immigration and psychopathology. In I. Al-Issa, and M. Tousignant (Eds.), *Ethnicity, immigration and psychopathology* (pp. 3-15). New York: Plenum.

Allen, R., Cushman, L. F., Morris, S., Feldman, J., Wade, C., McMahon, D. et al. (2000). Use of complementary and alternative medicine among Dominican emergency department patients. *American Journal of Emergency Medicine, 18*(1), 51-54.

Alva, S. A., & Jones, M. (1994). Psychosocial adjustment and self-reported patterns among Hispanics adolescents. *Journal of Early Adolescence, 14*, 432-448.

Anyon, J. (1997). *Ghetto schooling: a political economy of urban educational reform.* New York: Teacher's College.

Baez, A. (in press). Dominicans. In M. G. R. Gonzalez (Ed.), *Clinical practice with new Hispanic immigrants.* New York.

Baez, A., & Hernandez, D. (2001). Complementary spiritual beliefs in the Latino community: the interface with psychotherapy. *American Journal of Orthopsychiatry, 71*(4), 408-415.

Bentacourt, H., & Lopez, S. (1993). The study of culture ethnicity and race in American psychology. *American Psychologist, 48*, 629-637.

Bettes, B. A., Dusenbury, L., Kerner, J., & James-Ortiz, S. (1990). Ethnicity and psychosocial factors in alcohol and tobacco use in adolescence. *Child Development, 61*(2), 557-565.

Black, S. A., & Markides, K. S. (1994). Aging and generational patterns of alcohol consumption among Mexican Americans, Cuban Americans and mainland Puerto Ricans. *International Journal of Aging and Human Development, 39*(2), 97-103.

Caetano, R., & Clark, C. L. (1999). Trends and situational norms and attitude towards drinking among whites, blacks and hispanics:1984-1995. *Drug and Alcohol Dependence, 54*, 45-56.

Caetano, R., Clark, C. L., & Tam, T. (1998). Alcohol consumption among racial/ethnic minority: theory and research. *Alcohol Health and Research World, 22*(4), 233-241.

Canino, G. (1994). Alcohol use and misuse among Hispanic women: selected factors, processes, and studies. *International Journal of the Addictions, 29*(9), 1083-1100.

Canino, G. J., Burnam, A., & Caetano, R. (1992). The prevalence of alcohol abuse and/or dependence in two Hispanic communities. In J. E. Helzer, and G. J. Canino (Eds.), *Alcoholism in North America, Europe, and Asia* (pp. 131-158). New York: Oxford University Press.

Castro, M. J., & Boswell, T. D. (2002). The Dominican Diaspora Revisited: Dominicans and Dominican-American in a New Century. A North-South Agenda Paper.

Chapman, F. (1997). The Dominican Racial Setting: Frame of Reference for the Understanding of Cultural Diversity in the Dominican Republic. Occasional Paper No. 38.

Cosgrove, J. (1992). Remigration: the Dominican experience. *Social Development Issues, 14*(2/3), 101-120.

D'Imperio, R. L., Dubow, E. F., & Ippolito, M. F. (2000). Resilient and stress-affected adolescents in an urban setting. *Journal of Clinical Child Psychology, 29*(1), 129-142.

Drohan, D. A., Perez, O. M., Khan, A., Sullivan, A. N., Amaro, H., & Samet, J. H. (1997). Alcoholism in Latinos in the U.S.: Prevalence and screening. *JGIM, 12*(Suppl. 1), 124.

Duany, J. (1994). *Quisqueya on the Hudson: the transnational identity of Dominicans in Washington Heights. New York, CUNY Dominican Studies Institute.*

Dusenbury, L., Epstein, J. A., Botvin, G. J., & Diaz, T. (1994). Social influence predictors of alcohol use among New York Latino youth. *Addictive Behaviors, 19*(4), 363-372.

Epstein, J. A., Botvin, G. J., & Diaz, T. (2001). Alcohol use among Dominican and Puerto Rican adolescents residing in New York City: Role of Hispanic group and gender. *Developmental and Behavioral Pediatrics, 22*(2), 113-118.

Falicov, C. J. (1999). Religion and spiritual folk traditions in immigrant families: Therapeutic resources with Latinos. In B. Carter, and M. McGoldrick (Eds.), *The expanded family life cycle* (pp. 141-167). Boston: Allyn & Bacon.

Georges, E. (1989). *The making of a transnational community: migration, development and cultural changes in the Dominican Republic.* New York: Columbia University Press.

Gilbert, J. (1987). Alcohol consumption patterns in immigrant and later generation Mexican-American women. *Hispanic Journal of Behavioral Sciences, 9*(3), 299-317.

Gilbert, M. J., & Cervantes, R. C. (1986). Patterns and practices of alcohol use among Mexican-Americans: a comprehensive review. *Hispanic Journal of Behavioral Sciences, 8,* 1-60.

Gordis, E. (1999). *Are women more vulnerable to alcohol's effects?* National Institute on Alcohol Abuse and Alcoholism.

Gordon, A. J. (1978). Hispanic drinking after migration: the case of Dominican. *Medical Anthropology, 2*(4), 61-84.

Grasmuck, S., & Pessar, P. R. (1991). *Between two islands: Dominican international migration.* Berkeley, CA: University of California Press.

Greenfield, T. K., & Room, R. (1997). Situational norms for drinking and drunkenness: trends in the U.S. adult population, 1979-1990. *Addiction, 92,* 33-47.

Hernandez, R., & Torres Saillant, S. (1997). *Constructing the New York Area Hispanic mosaic: a demographic portrait of Colombians and Dominicans in New York minorities, education, empowerment.* CA: NALEO Educational Fund.

Iltis, C. E. (2002). Adult Dominicans in therapy: psychotherapists' perceptions of cultural treatment issues. *Dissertation Abstracts International: Section B: The Sciences and Engineering, 62*(11-B), 5377.

Kail, B., Zayas, L. H., & Malgady, R. G. (2000). Depression, acculturation, and motivations for alcohol use among young Colombian, Dominican, and Puerto Rican men. *Hispanic Journal of Behavioral Sciences, 22*(1), 64-77.

La Roche, M. J. (1999). The association of social relations and depression levels among Dominicans in the United States. *Hispanic Journal of Behavioral Sciences, 21*(4), 420-430.

Lee, D. J., Markides, K. S., & Ray, L. A. (1997). Epidemiology of self-reported past heavy drinking in Hispanic adults. *Ethnicity and Health, 2*(1-2), 77-88.

Logan, J. R. (2001). *The New Latinos: who they are, where they are.* Lewis Mumford Center for Comparative Urban and Regional Research.

Lopez, N. (2002). Rewriting race and gender high school lessons: second-generation Dominicans in New York City. *Teachers College Record, 104*(6), 1187-1203.

Nielsen, A. L. F., J.A. (2001). Drinking patterns among Hispanic adolescents: results from a national survey. *Journal of Studies on Alcohol, 62*(4), 448-456.

Ojito, M. (1997). Dominicans, scrabbling for hope: as poverty rises more women head the households. *New York Times*, p. 1.

Oostveen, T., Knibbe, R., & DeVries, H. (1996). Social influences on young adults' alcohol consumption: norms, modeling, pressure, socializing and conformity. *Addictive Behaviors, 21*, 187-197.

Phinney, J. S. (1996). When we talk about American ethnic groups what do we mean? *American Psychologist, 51*(9), 918-927.

Randolph, W. M., Stroup Benham, C., Black, S. A., & Markides, K. S. (1998). Alcohol use among Cuban-Americans, Mexican-Americans, and Puerto Ricans. *Alcohol Health and Research World, 22*(4), 265-269.

Rohther, L. (1998). Island life not idyllic for youths from U.S. *New York Times*, p. 4.

SAMSHA, S. A. a. M. H. S. A. (1999). Hispanics in substance abuse treatment. *The DASIS Report*.

Sontag, M. G., & Dugger, C. W. (1998). The new immigrant tie: a shuttle between worlds. *New York Times*.

Sorlie, P. D., Backland, E., Johnson, N. J., & Rogot, E. (1993). Mortality by Hispanic status in the United States. *Journal of the American Medical Association, 270*(20), 2446-2468.

Torres-Saillant, S., & Hernandez, R. (1998). *The Dominican Americans. The new Americans series*.

U.S. Bureau of the Census. (2000). Washington, D.C.: U.S. Government Printing Office.

Wells, K., Klap, R., Koike, A., & Sherbourne, C. (2001). Ethnic disparities in unmet need for alcoholism, drug abuse, and mental health care. *American Journal of Psychiatry, 158*(12), 2027-2032.

Westhoff, W., McDermott, R. J., & Holcomb, D. R. (1996). HIV risk behaviors: a comparison of U.S. Hispanics and Dominican Republic youth. *AIDS Education and Prevention, 8*(2), 106-114.

Zayas, L. H. (1992). Childrearing, social stress, and child abuse: clinical considerations with Hispanic families. *Journal of Social Distress and the Homeless, 1*, 291-309.

Zayas, L. H., Rojas, M., & Malgady, R. G. (1998). Alcohol and drug use, and depression among Hispanic men in early adulthood. *American Journal of Community Psychology, 26*(3), 425-438.

Chapter 5

# Onset of Alcohol and Other Drug Use Among Latino Gang Members: A Preliminary Analysis

Mario De La Rosa, PhD
Douglas Rugh, MSW

**SUMMARY.** Recent information from epidemiological studies of alcohol and other drug use among gang members has documented that alcohol and other drug use is a serious problem among Latino gang members. Despite the extensive body of research on the onset of alcohol and other drug use among high-risk adolescents and the drug-using behaviors of gang members, particularly Latino gang members, there is a limited amount of research on the onset of alcohol and other drug-using behaviors among Latino gang members. The study described in this paper explores the patterns of alcohol and drug use initiation among male Latino gang members. Data presented in this report is from a preliminary

Mario De La Rosa is Associate Professor, and Douglas Rugh is a doctoral candidate, Florida International University, School of Social Work, University Park, ECS 463, 11200 SW 8th Street, Miami, FL 33199.

This research project was supported by a National Institute on Drug Abuse grant (S R24 DA 12203). The opinions expressed herein are those of the authors and do not necessarily reflect the opinions or official policy of the National Institute on Drug Abuse or any part of the U.S. Department of Health and Human Services.

[Haworth co-indexing entry note]: "Onset of Alcohol and Other Drug Use Among Latino Gang Members: A Preliminary Analysis." De La Rosa, Mario, and Douglas Rugh. Co-published simultaneously in *Alcoholism Treatment Quarterly* (The Haworth Press, Inc.) Vol. 23, No. 2/3, 2005, pp. 67-85; and: *Latinos and Alcohol Use/Abuse Revisited: Advances and Challenges for Prevention and Treatment Programs* (ed: Melvin Delgado) The Haworth Press, Inc., 2005, pp. 67-85. Single or multiple copies of this article are available for a fee from The Haworth Document Delivery Service [1-800-HAWORTH, 9:00 a.m. - 5:00 p.m. (EST). E-mail address: docdelivery@haworthpress.com].

Available online at http://www.haworthpress.com/web/ATQ
doi:10.1300/J020v23n02_05

analysis of 40 male gang members from a larger study of 81 male gang members. This preliminary analysis suggests important age and drug of choice differences between Latino gang members and other populations. Understanding the differences will assist in developing more effective programs to prevent the onset of alcohol and other drug use among Latino adolescent gang members. *[Article copies available for a fee from The Haworth Document Delivery Service: 1-800-HAWORTH. E-mail address: <docdelivery@haworthpress.com> Website: <http://www.HaworthPress. com> © 2005 by The Haworth Press, Inc. All rights reserved.]*

**KEYWORDS.** Latinos, alcohol, gangs

## INTRODUCTION

Investigations into alcohol and other drug use behaviors of gang members and the onset of alcohol and other drug use[1] among high-risk adolescents[2] have received considerable attention by social scientists during the past fifteen years (e.g., DeWit, Offord, & Wong, 1997; Hunt & Laidler, 2001; Kandel & Faust, 1975; Kandel & Yamaguchi, 1993; Labouvie, Bates, & Pandina, 1997; Stewart, Brown, & Myers, 1997). One clear result from this research is that there are early behavioral differences between low at risk[3] and high at risk groups. High at risk groups begin to use alcohol and other drugs earlier and with greater frequency than low-risk groups. Furthermore, high at risk adolescents are more likely to join gangs, which greatly increase the likelihood of initiation and rapid progression toward illicit drug use. Even though these fundamental processes are recognized, alcohol and other drug use and gang activity continue to escalate (Egley, 2000; Hegan, Carley, & Strickler, 2001). In order to develop a better understanding of the processes related to high at risk adolescents and gang membership, scientists have begun to look at ethnic differences in the developmental course of alcohol and other drug use. Comparative research suggests diverse etiologic pathways to alcohol and drug use across ethnic groups (Guerra, Romano, Samuels, & Kass, 2000; Stewart et al., 1997). So if a particular ethnic group can be identified as high risk, then an opportunity arises for a detailed study of the factors associated with the onset of alcohol and other drug use.

Recent information about alcohol and other drug use among gang members reveals a high number of gangs within Latino communities (Romero, 2001; Vigil, 2000). Despite the extensive body of research on the onset of alcohol and other drug use among high-risk adolescents and the drug-using behaviors of gang members, particularly Latino gang members, there is little research on the factors associated with the onset of alcohol and other drug use behaviors among Latino gang members (Guerra et al., 2000). The study described in this manuscript explores the social factors associated with the onset of alcohol and other drug use among Latino gang members.

The purpose of this manuscript, therefore, is to augment the research literature by presenting information from an ethnographic study that collected information on the onset of alcohol and other drug use among a cohort of 40 Latino, mostly Puerto Rican, gang members living in Lawrence, Massachusetts, a small city in Northeast United States. Descriptive data is presented on age of onset of alcohol and other drug use behaviors, types of drug first used, the settings of first use, and the group they were a part of at the time of first use. The data provides much needed information on the onset of alcohol and other drug use among Latino gang members. Additionally, the results can be utilized as the foundation of future epidemiological studies regarding the patterns of alcohol and other drug use among Latino and non-Latino gang members and other populations high at risk for alcohol and other drug use or dependency.

## REVIEW OF LITERATURE

During the past fifteen years, research regarding the onset of alcohol and other drug use among high-risk American adolescents and drug-using behaviors of gang members follow similar paths but divergent methodological approaches in their collection of data on the drug-using behaviors of adolescents (De La Rosa, Segal, & Lopez, 1999). Similar paths because researchers in each of these two areas of drug use research search for patterns of drug use among adolescents high at risk for using and abusing drugs and alcohol. Divergent methodological approaches because researchers exploring the onset of alcohol and other drug use among high at risk American adolescents have used cross-sectional surveys while those investigating alcohol and other drug use among gang members have used ethnographic methods. Often the findings from cross-sectional surveys have been based on data collected from adolescents incarcerated in juvenile detention centers or drug treatment programs. In contrast, findings from ethnographic surveys have been based on data collected from street-based ethnographic methods. Included below is a review of these two areas of research with a special emphasis on results from studies that focus on the alcohol and other drug-using behaviors of Latino gang members.

## Onset of Alcohol and Other Drug Use Among High at Risk Adolescents

Research regarding the onset of alcohol and other drug use among high at risk adolescents has its foundation in the seminal work of Kandel and Faust (1975) stages in adolescent involvement in alcohol and other drug use. They established that adolescents' onset of drug use typically begins with alcohol or cigarette use progressing to marijuana and other illicit drug use. Furthermore, adolescents are unlikely to experiment with marijuana without prior use of alcohol or cigarettes, and very few adolescents try hard drugs without prior use of marijuana. Other studies have also demonstrated that use of various drugs shows a sequential pattern in adolescence consistent with Kandel's four-stage model (Elliott, Huizinga, & Menard, 1989; Hops, Tidelsley, Lichtenstein, Ary, & Sherman, 1990). The stages of drug initiation suggest that adolescents' experience with different drugs occur at different ages.

Findings from national studies support the idea that different ages are associated with different drugs. For the general population, the highest probability for the onset of alcohol and marijuana use is approximately 18 years of age and the highest probability for the onset of cocaine is two years later while for high-risk youth the highest probability for the onset of marijuana use is 15 and for cocaine use is 19 (Wagner & Anthony, 2002). Findings from smaller studies support the idea that a group of high-risk adolescents begin using alcohol and drugs earlier than the general population. For the high at risk adolescent, alcohol use begins around the age of 12 (DeWit et al., 1997). The results from this research suggest that at 12 years of age, a family member or a close relation with the family often introduces the adolescent to alcohol within the home. Once an individual enters adolescence, friends and peers begin to play a significant role in introducing and maintaining their involvement in alcohol and drug-using behaviors.

Besides population patterns of behavior, important individual differences began to emerge. As Kandel and colleagues acknowledge (Kandel & Yamaguchi, 1993), adolescents vary in their patterns of alcohol and other drug use even though they go through broadly comparable phases of use at roughly the same ages. For example, although many adolescents engage in experimental use of substances, only some go on to develop serious alcohol and other drug use problems in adolescence or adulthood. Johnston, O'Malley, and Bachman (1989) demonstrated that only a subgroup of adolescents in a national sample of high school students showed a strong upward trend in their intensity of alcohol and other drug use, whereas a substantial group of adolescent alcohol and other drug users engage only in minimal experimentation with substances. Of those who do go on to develop more serious alcohol and other drug use problems, the majority are male. Males also tend to use different drugs from females and with greater frequency (DeWit et al., 1997; Kandel & Yamaguchi, 1993).

Recent research also emphasizes the importance of individual differences in the way adolescents progress through the four-stage model described by (Kandel & Faust, 1975). For example, a panel study of 764 students measured in sixth, eighth, and tenth grades found four distinct patterns of escalation in alcohol and other drug use over time. Although Kandel's model applies reasonably well, the time of initiation and rates of progression vary widely within these groups (Zapert, Snow, & Tebes, 2002). Further studies report that the type of drug chosen for initiation directly affects the drug use trajectories and use of other types of drugs. This progressive relationship was shown with alcohol, cigarettes, and marijuana. Cigarette use, in particular, was particularly important in the subsequent involvement of alcohol and marijuana (Duncan, Duncan, & Hops, 1998). Basically, increased involvement with legal drugs constitutes an important step in the transition to hard drug use for most adolescents. This association was further demonstrated between different classes of drugs and across different ethnic groups. Weekly alcohol use followed marijuana use and preceded use of all other illicit drugs for Hispanic, White, and Black youth. However, for Asians, alcohol use follows use of hard drugs. Weekly smoking formed a distinct stage between initial use of pills and other hard drugs for non-Latino Whites (Ellickson, Hays, & Bell, 1992). Guerra et al. (2000) used data from the 1996 Youth Risk Behavior Survey to analyze ethnic differences in the progression from licit to illicit drug use. They reported that progression was significantly associated with Black ethnicity and male sex. Breaches in the sequence (i.e., use of illicit substances before licit substances) were more likely to occur for Black male and Latino female youth, compared to White youth, when the analyses controlled for maternal education. These differences between gender and ethnicity challenge underlying assumptions about alcohol and other drug use initiation.

Despite the growing body of research on the onset of alcohol and other drug use among high-risk adolescents, research rarely involves the collection of data on the onset of alcohol and other drug use among adolescents involved in gangs. Furthermore, with few exceptions (e.g., Guerra et al., 2000) this research focuses on collecting information on the onset of alcohol and other drug use among White non-Latino adolescents. The findings reported in this manuscript seek to address this gap in alcohol and other drug use research literature by documenting the onset of alcohol and other drug use among Latino gang members. This is important because we know that membership in a gang is a primary risk factor for later alcohol and other drug use problems (Esbensen & Winfree, 1998; Huff, 1998; Thornberry & Burch, 1997), and we also know that a large number of gangs are formed in Latino communities (Romero, 2001; Vigil, 2000).

## Epidemiological Research on Alcohol and Other Drug Use Among Latino Gang Members

The interest in exploring the drug-using behaviors of Latino gangs has it roots with the development of the cocaine and crack trade during the beginning of the 1980s and the reported involvement of Latino gangs in this trade. Prior to 1990, research on Latino gangs concentrated on the reasons Latino gangs form and the role that these gangs played in the lives of their members (De La Rosa & Caris, 1993). This research found that Hispanic gangs often supplied emotional and financial support and protection to gang members that was lacking in their families (Moore, 1978; Moore, Vigil, & Garcia, 1983; Vigil, 1988). Drug use, dealing, and drug-related violence was not the primary focus of these studies. In part, this was due to the fact that during the 1970s drug use and dealing by Latino gang members was mostly an individual or small-group behavior, which was frequently not sanctioned or known by other gang members or leaders (Moore, 1978). Similarly this early research did not study differences in Latino gangs based on ethnicity or explore the effect of community institutions and agencies on gang members' behaviors (De La Rosa & Caris, 1993).

With the development of the crack trade in the late '80s and early '90s, data became available that linked Latino gangs to the drug trade. Since then there has been a growing interest in examining drug use and dealing and drug-related violence in gangs in more depth. For instance, a strong relationship between drug dealing and violence among Mexican-American gangs in San Francisco that were involved in the crack trade was found (Waldorf, 1993). Another study examined the involvement of established Puerto Rican gangs in the crack trade and found that the opportunities provided by the crack trade created a drug dealing subculture within established Puerto Rican gangs in Milwaukee (Moore & Hagedorn, 1996). As part of this study, Moore and Hagedorn also report that while many of these gangs were formed initially to provide a network of support and protection for their members, the crack trade and the lack of economic opportunities in Milwaukee had turned them into criminal enterprises. In interviews with gang members, many members preferred to have a good paying job in the legal economy but had turned to the crack trade out of economic necessity (Moore & Hagedorn, 1996). The data from Milwaukee corroborates the strong relationship between drug use, drug dealing, and violence found among Latino gang and non-Latino gangs in other studies. The conclusion from both of these studies is that those gang members, who were drug users and were more deeply involved in the drug trade, were more likely to be involved in violent incidents than gang members who did not use or deal drugs.

Besides drug dealing, researchers have begun to investigate alcohol and other drug use within gangs. Valdez (1996) found that Mexican-American adolescents who joined gangs with a prior history of drug use, often intensified their drug use after becoming gang members. Other researchers have reported similar findings. In general, the findings indicate that youth who become members of gangs use more drugs than before they were members and while they are members, they use more drugs then after they leave the gang (Esbensen & Winfree, 1998; Huff, 1998; Thornberry & Burch, 1997). Not only does gang membership appear to facilitate drug use in those individuals who were abusing drugs before becoming a member but also the vast majority of gang members use drugs.

Despite this growing body of research there continues to be a dearth of research on the drug-using behaviors of gang members and the role gangs play in exacerbating the development of drug use, abuse, and dependency among Latino gang members. Most needed is research on drug-using trajectories of Latino gang members including the onset of drug use and the social context in which such onset of drug use occurs with adolescents who go on to become gang members. The results presented in this manuscript provide one of the first studies that have examined the onset of alcohol and other drug use among Latino gangs and can serve as the foundation for the development of future research on this topic.

## METHODOLOGY AND SOURCES OF DATA

The interpretations presented here draw on observation and extensive fieldwork over a number of years, specifically on data from 2001 and 2002. The site of the study was Lawrence, Massachusetts, a small city (pop. 70,207) in the east of the United States located about forty minutes from a major metropolitan area. Lawrence has a high concentration of Latino residents, mostly of Puerto Rican and Dominican descent. The city, known in the area as the "Immigrant City," is predominantly home to a minority of third to sixth generation immigrants of varying ethnic backgrounds and a majority of first and second generation Latinos: Puerto Rican and newcomers from the Dominican Republic, Cuba and several other distinct cultures from Central America. The population of Lawrence has undergone a dramatic shift in 15 years, with a growth of Latino residents from 16 percent to 42 percent from the 1980 to the 1990 census. Lawrence's Latino population is also extraordinarily young, resulting in one of the highest proportions of population under 5 and under 18 in Massachusetts. It is one the most economically depressed communities in the state of Massachusetts with poverty rates consistently higher than the rest of the state (Jaysane, 2002).

Latino gang members interviewed were recruited from neighborhoods thought to have a high concentration of gang members. The research follows a collaborative model (cf. Moore, 1978), in which gang members cooperate with academic staff to focus the research design and construct interview schedules. Before the identification and recruitment of gang members, the staff of the project (community researchers) spent time in each neighborhood getting to know people who live there, observing neighborhood activities, assessing neighborhood safety and receptivity to being studied and determining whether emerging gangs are present. The staff ranked each neighborhood on the basis of safety, accessibility and presence of gangs. The neighborhoods that ranked highest across these criteria were selected for the study.

### Excerpts

Community researchers spent extensive time in the selected neighborhoods acquiring the trust needed to gain access. One method that community researchers used to develop such trust was to volunteer to help with various neighborhoods activities (e.g., volunteer to coach basketball at the local recreational center, assist gang members in obtaining social, health and job-related services, etc.). In addition to getting to know gang members, community researchers also developed friend-ships with major gatekeepers in the neighborhoods.

The interviews took place using "ethnographically driven targeted sampling." Once community researchers became familiar with the neighborhoods, they began to talk with community gatekeepers to de-termine where gang members congregate and began to develop a roster of active gang members that they could approach for interviews. The gang members whom the community researchers had a good rapport with were approached first. In asking a gang member to participate in the project, the community researcher made it clear that their participa-tion was voluntary and all information that was collected would be con-fidential.

Gang members were interviewed at the community field office or on the street. Only one gang member was interviewed at one time in order to preserve confidentiality and avoid confrontations between members of rival gangs. Those gang members who agreed to be interviewed were interviewed on the spot if they agreed to do so or an appointment was made for a later time in a place they felt comfortable. They were also asked if the interview could be tape recorded. None of the gang members refused to be recorded and therefore all the interviews were tape re-corded. The interviews lasted about 2 hours, and the community re-searcher also took notes during the interview. Gang members were paid $50 for their participation at the end of the interview. To safeguard the confidentiality of the data each gang member was assigned a number at the beginning of the interview.

## Data Transcription and Analysis

Several steps were taken to transcribe the data. Three research staff-persons were involved in the process. Since the data were collected both in Spanish and English, one research staff worked only on the transcrip-tion of the English interviews, while the other two staff persons were re-sponsible for transcribing the Spanish interviews. Initially, Spanish interviews were supposed to be translated from Spanish into English for purposes of analysis. This strategy was reworked once the research staff had a sense of the extensive amount of time involved in translation and back translation of the interviews (approximately 90-minute tape inter-view took approximately 40 hours to complete). Due to limited project resources and time, it was decided to store the data in Spanish. Atlas.ti software made it possible to keep transcripts in their original form and proceed with coding in English. Other projects may have a difficult time approaching transcriptions and coding in this way if the staff is not bi-lingual. For instance, if the analysis is to be done by a person not fluent in the language needed, then this option is not available and it becomes necessary to invest resources in translation and back translation.

Entering the data into Atlas.ti was a twofold process. Two Herme-neutic Units were created, a Spanish and English data file. This allowed staff to begin preliminary coding of the data. Since not all three staff in-volved in the preliminary coding were fluent in both languages, this separation was necessary. Before the Atlas.ti software could be used to analyze the collected information, a coding scheme was developed as a guide. After preliminary reading of ten randomly selected transcripts by the project staff, a coding scheme based on a person's drug use trajec-tory was developed to analyze the alcohol and other drug use data. Each stage of development (i.e., initiation, progression, addiction, treatment and remission) was used as super categories and entered into Atlas.ti for analysis.

The initial data that emerged led to the further development of subcate-gories within each of the alcohol and other drug use super categories. For drug use initiation, which is the data reported in this manuscript, textual analysis revealed four subcategories: age, who else was involved, type of drug, and the location of drug onset. The results of this analysis follow.

## RESULTS

### Sample

The staff conducted interviews with 81 active male gang members: Sixty-seven (83%) of the gang members were Puerto Rican, 9 (11%) were Dominican, and the remaining 5 (6%) were other Latino or un-known. The youngest gang member interviewed was 18 and the oldest was 48 years old; 20 (25%) of the gang members were between the ages of 18 and 21, 30 (37%) were between the ages of 21 and 30 years old, 14 (17%) were over the age of 30 years old, and the remaining 17 gang members' age is unknown. The majority of those interviewed belong to three gangs: the Latin Gangster Disciples, Latin Kings, and Neta and the rest to other smaller gangs like the Outlaws, Crips, LTS, Got Life, Im-mature Kids, Castillos Allegres, and Stables. Data presented in this re-port is from a preliminary analysis of 40 of the 81 gang members interviewed and includes textual data from the interviews to highlight the context in which the onset of drug use occurred. The focus of this analysis is on the patterns of alcohol and other drug use onset.

## Onset of Alcohol and Other Drug Use

*Age of alcohol or drug use onset?* The average age of onset is 11 years old with 46% starting before the age of 11 with a range between the ages of 5 and 16 years. The textual data presented below highlights how young some of these gang members were when they first used drugs and the context in which such use occurred.

Excerpt 1

Q: When you were 7 or 8 years old, you had smoked cigarettes. What other drugs did you experiment with?
R: Smoking weed. I used to go to Penn's Pharmacy and I used to steal Pampers for one of the gang leaders. . . . He used to be like I'll give two, three joints, for you to go get me some Pampers. Buck and a couple of the fellows, we used to go get Pampers. He'd give us a joint or two.

Excerpt 2

Q: Can you tell me the first time you use drugs, drank, or smoke?
R: The first time I was eleven years old. I got so drunk. I remember they bought a case of Colt.
Q: Who's they?
R: It was the people I used to hang around we went to the train tracks. We got so drunk.

Excerpt 3

Q: Can you tell me the first time you tried anything?
R: It was nine or ten, nine, the cigarettes. The older guys say here, you could smoke, it ain't nothing . . . I remember only doing a drag. I didn't like it at all. I coughed. It was nasty to me.

*Who they were with during the onset of alcohol or drug use?* Twenty-four (60%) of the gang members reported that they were with friends when they first started to use and 7 (18%) reported that they were with family members. The remaining 9 (23%) gang members reported that they were either with other gang members or alone. Among the family members, uncles and stepfathers were among the ones most frequently identified. The important role that friends play in the onset of drug use is highlighted in the excerpts below and above.

Q:   Tell me about the first time you smoked a cigarette.
R:   Well, it was me and my friend Buck and there was a whole bunch of us. We were called the Dynamite Kids. At that age, I was a 'wanna-be.' I wanted to be like the older gang members and there was a few of us. There was about eight, nine of us that were the way that I was, not going to school and just hanging out in the streets. We would just walk around and we'd see cigarettes on the ground or somebody threw a cigarette on the floor cause we seen the older guys smoking. We'll pick it up and smoke. We'll get a head rush and be like, yeah, this where it's at.

Family members also had a significant impact in the onset of drug use behavior among the gang members interviewed as depicted in the excerpts below.

Excerpt 1

Q:   Tell me about the first time you used drugs.
R:   I think I had with my aunt, my family. Everything I did I did with my family. They will drink, I will drink, they will smoke weed, I will smoke weed . . .

Excerpt 2

Q:   Now tell about the first time you smoked weed (marijuana was the first drug of choice use by this gang member).
R:   Yeah, it was with my uncle. I remember it was uncle Joey.
Q:   Tell me about?
R:   I was in grandmother's house and he was in the room. I don't know, when you are a little kid, you are nosey, especially with your uncle. You're always going to look up to your uncle. I was being nosey and went I went in the room. I can see my uncle and he grabbed and goes, you wanna try this.

*Where was the first drug used?* Fifteen (38%) of the gang members reported that they were on the street when they first used, which included alleys, parks, and street corners, while 13 (33%) reported that they were in their parent's home, which was most often the mother's home, and 5 (13%) reported that were in or around school grounds. The remaining 7 (18%) gang members did not discuss where they first used drugs. Not surprisingly, the family home was the second most common place where the gang members interviewed started their drug use. Two excerpts from the gang members interviewed shows just how comfortable some of the gang member felt using drugs in their home during their first drug use.

Excerpt 1

Q: OK, could you talk to me about the first time you used drugs, where were you?
R: At the back yard of mom's house. At the backyard they can't see us. The window is in the front. The back there is a window but my mom don't live in the back. My mom lives in the front.

Excerpt 2

Q: [The response is in relation to a question the interviewer asked the gang member earlier on in the interview where he first used drugs.]
R: It was outside the home . . . I took my first sip I believe it was in the sweet sixteenth party of my sister. One of my mom's friends sent me to the kitchen to get him another beer and his beer still like had a quarter in it. So I took a swig of beer and I didn't like the taste.

*First type of drug ever used?* Eighteen (45%) of the gang members reported that they used alcohol first. This was followed by 13 (33%) gang members who reported that they used marijuana and 9 (23%) who said that they started with cigarettes. Of those who reported marijuana as their first drug, approximately 9 started to smoke prior to the age of 14 years old. Furthermore, 11 of the gang members who said that their drug use started with marijuana used other illicit drugs. The most frequently cited illicit drug used was heroin 6 (55%) followed by cocaine 5 (45%) (see Figure 1). Regarding alcohol use by the gang members, an example of extremely early memories of drinking as an infant is discussed by one of the gang members below.

FIGURE 1. Use of Other Illicit Drugs by Marijuana Users (n = 11)

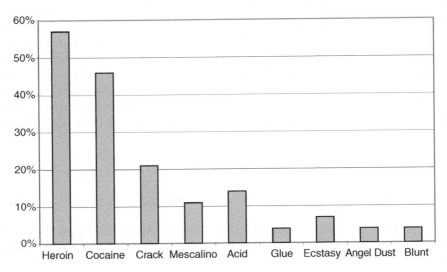

Q:  Do you remember the first time you drank?
R:  Oh yeah, I was young. I was like four or five years old. I would al-
    ways be up cause I was a hyper person. I was real hyper. I was a
    bad little kid. Like they would always tell me I was a bad little kid
    and I was hyper. I was always in and out of things, where I wasn't
    supposed to be. So to knock me out, they'd give me a sip, give me
    two, three sips of beers. I'll fall asleep real quick. I believe that's
    why I became an addict and an alcoholic. I believe that truly.

Regarding, the use of marijuana as the first drug of choice ever used,
the gang members reported such use at a slightly older age than those
whose onset of drug use began with the use of alcohol. Nevertheless,
many of the gang members whose onset of drug use began with the use
of marijuana started at a relatively young age as exemplified in the information gathered from two of the gang interviewers below.

Excerpt 1

Q:  What did you do when you first started using drugs?
R:  I smoked my first blunt. It was a joint. I was thirteen. I felt
    good. Got high and sick. Hanging out with my friends.

Excerpt 2

Q: Before we can talking about Lawrence tell me about the first time you used drugs?

R: The first time on used drugs I smoked marijuana was when I was in New York. I was twelve. I remember hanging out on the train. There was guys sniffing glue in a bag. Back in those days it was the glue bag sniffing glue. I never liked that.

## Discussion of Results

The study reported in this paper suggests that both similar and divergent patterns of alcohol and other drug use exist between the general population and Latino gang members. This study supports the notion that adolescents initiate alcohol and drug use with family and peers. Another similar finding is that the majority of the adolescents used alcohol or drugs in their parents' home or on the streets. In addition to the similarities, the study also suggests differences associated with Latino gang members. The findings suggest that Latino gang members begin to use alcohol or marijuana earlier than adolescents in the general population. Not only do Latino gang members initiate drug use earlier, but also there are some indications that some adolescents begin with marijuana not alcohol or cigarettes.

In this analysis, gang members who started with marijuana also reported a number of illicit drug use in later years as shown in Figure 1. While it is impossible to determine from this data whether there is a significant pattern of progression to more serious drugs by adolescents who begin drug use with marijuana, additional research will be able to determine the implications of starting with marijuana. Further research is also needed to determine the contextual factors, such as poverty and living in crime-ridden neighborhoods, which play a significant role in the initiation of alcohol and other drug use among gang members.

Additionally, the results suggest that a significant number of gang members (14 out of 40) remain actively involved with the gang beyond the age of 30, which seems to be higher than that reported in previous research on Latino gang members. Whether the older age of some of the gang members in this study is an artifact of the data collection activities of the study or due to factors associated with living within in a small city needs to be further investigated.

## LIMITATIONS OF THE STUDY

Since this is a preliminary report, the researchers limited the inferences. For example, one area for further exploration is the onset of drug use with marijuana as opposed to alcohol. A more complete analysis will provide a better understanding of the onset of drug use among this population. Additionally, because of the inherent difficulties in gaining access to this population, the 40 gang members interviewed in this study may not be representative of Latino gang members in the city of Lawrence or elsewhere, thus limiting the generalizabilty of this study findings. Furthermore, since the study's primary focus was documenting the drug-using behaviors of Latino male gangs members, the study's findings are not applicable on the onset of alcohol and other drug use among Latino female gang members. Future research should document the drug-using behaviors of Latino female gang members. Finally, since the collection of data from gang members was based upon self-reports, the possibility exists that some of the interviewed gang members distorted their drug behaviors, calling to question the validity of the collected information.

## CONCLUSION

The study is one of the first studies that have documented the onset of alcohol and other drug use among Latino gang members living in a small city environment allowing the findings to be compared with previous research on the drug-using behaviors of Latino gang members living in large urban areas. It provides further evidence that the drug use trajectories of gang members may differ from adolescents not involved in gangs, prompting the need for additional studies in this area of drug use research. Additionally, the importance of friends and family members in the onset of alcohol and other drug use in this study sample corroborates previous research on this topic among U.S. adolescents, but also highlights the need for additional research that will document the role of community level factors (e.g., poverty, availability of drugs) in the onset of alcohol and other drug use among adolescents. Further, this study provides additional evidence that earlier onset of alcohol and other drug use is associated with involvement with other drugs and possible progression to substance use behaviors.

The study has several implications for prevention. The results provide evidence that drug use prevention interventions programs should target Latino adolescents at risk of using drugs during their early child-hood years. The results also reinforce the importance of involving Latino families as a strategy to prevent drug use among Latino adolescents. Efforts also need to be redoubled to create innovative peer-based drug use prevention that will target Latino adolescents who have joined gangs as an alternative to their gang lifestyles. In summary, this study may open new avenues for developing interventions with greater specificity in relation to Latino gang members' alcohol and other drug use. These approaches may compliment existing universal strategies to prevent adolescent alcohol and other drug use.

## NOTES

1. The term "other drug use" refers to the use of illicit drugs such as marijuana, cocaine, heroin.
2. The term "high at risk adolescent" refers to youth who have been adjudicated as juvenile delinquents, come from families where there is a history of drug use or child use, are experiencing academic problems, or have dropped out of school.
3. The term "low at risk" refers to the majority of youth and families who do not demonstrate overt alcohol and other drug use or legal problems. These youth are experiencing age appropriate problems; however, they appear to have the support necessary to successfully cope.

## REFERENCES

De La Rosa, M., & Caris, L. (1993). The Drugs/Crime Connection Among Hispanics: A Review of Current Research. In B. Kail, A. Sachez-Myers & D. Watts (Eds.), *Hispanics and Drug Use* (pp. 81-100): Charles Thomas Printing.

De La Rosa, M., Segal, B., & Lopez, R. (1999). Conducting Drug Use Research with Minority Populations: Advances and Issues. *Drugs and Society, 14*, 1-2.

DeWit, D. J., Offord, D. R., & Wong, M. (1997). Patterns of Onset and Cessation of Drug Use over the Early Part of the Life Course. *Health Education & Behavior, 24*(6), 746-758.

Duncan, S. C., Duncan, T. E., & Hops, H. (1998). Progression of Alcohol, Cigarette, and Marijuana Use in Adolescence. *Journal of Behavioral Medicine, 21*(4), 375-388.

Egley, A. (2000). *Highlights of the 1999 National Youth Gang Survey* (Fact Sheet 2000-20). Washington, D.C.: Department of Justice.

Ellickson, P. L., Hays, R. D., & Bell, R. M. (1992). Stepping Through the Drug Use Sequence: Longitudinal Scalogram Analysis of Initiation and Regular Use. *Journal of Abnormal Psychology, 101*(3), 441-451.

Elliott, D. S., Huizinga, D., & Menard, S. (1989). *Multiple Problem Youth: Delinquency, Alcohol and Other Drug Use, and Mental Health Problems*. New York: Springer.

Esbensen, F. A., & Winfree, L. T. (1998). Race and Gender Differences Between Gang and Non-gang Youth: Results from a Multi-site Survey. *Justice Quarterly, 15*(4), 505-526.

Guerra, L. M., Romano, P. S., Samuels, S. J., & Kass, P. H. (2000). Ethnic Differences in Adolescent Substance Initiation Sequences. *Archives of Pediatrics & Adolescent Medicine, 154*(11), 1089-1095.

Hegan, C., Carley, K., & Strickler, G. (2001). *Societal Cost of Substance Use, the Economic Cost of Substance Use to the US Economy* (Published Report): Schneider Institute for Health Policy.

Hops, H., Tidelsley, E., Lichtenstein, E., Ary, D., & Sherman, L. (1990). Parent-adolescent Problem-solving Interactions and Drug Use. *American Journal of Drug and Alcohol Use, 16*, 239-258.

Huff, C. R. (1998). *Criminal Behavior of Gang Members and At-risk Youths*. Washington, D.C.: U.S. Department of Justice.

Hunt, G. P., & Laidler, K. J. (2001). Alcohol and Violence in the Lives of Gang Members. *Alcohol Research & Health, 25*(1), 66-71.

Jaysane, A. P. (2002). *The Community Context of Health in Lawrence, Massachusetts*. Lawrence, MA: Merrimack College.

Johnston, L. D., O'Malley, P. M., & Bachman, J. G. (1989). *Drug Use, Drinking and Smoking: National Survey Results from High School, College, and Young Adult Populations 1975-1988*. Rockville, MD: National Institute on Drug Use.

Kandel, D., & Faust, R. (1975). Sequence and Stages in Patterns of Adolescent Drug Use. *Archives of General Psychiatry, 32*, 923-932.

Kandel, D., & Yamaguchi, K. (1993). From Beer to Crack: Developmental Patterns of Drug Involvement. *American Journal of Public Health, 83*(6), 851-855.

Labouvie, E., Bates, M. E., & Pandina, R. J. (1997). Age of First Use: Its Reliability and Predictive Utility. *Journal of Studies on Alcohol, 58*(6), 638-643.

Moore, J. W. (1978). *Homeboys: Gangs, Drugs, and Prison in the Barrios of Los Angeles*. Philadelphia: Temple University Press.

Moore, J. W., & Hagedorn, J. M. (1996). *Drugs, Posses, Gangs, and the Underclass in Milwaukee* (DA07128). Rockville, MD: National Institute on Drug Use.

Moore, J. W., Vigil, J. D., & Garcia, R. (1983). Residence and Territoriality in Chicano Gangs. *Social Problems, 31*, 182-194.

Romero, M. (2001). State Violence, and the Social and Legal Construction of Latino Criminality from El Bandido to Gang Member. *Denver University Law Review, 78*(4), 1081-1118.

Stewart, D. G., Brown, S. A., & Myers, M. G. (1997). Antisocial Behavior and Psychoactive Substance Involvement Among Hispanic and Non-Hispanic Caucasian Adolescents in Substance Use Treatment. *Journal of Child & Adolescent Substance Use, 6*(4), 1-22.

Thornberry, T. P., & Burch, J. H. (1997). *Gang Members and Delinquent Behavior* (165154). Washington, D.C.: U.S. Department of Justice.

Valdez, A. (1996). *Alcohol and Other Drug Use Among Mexican-American School-Age Youth* (DA 07234). Rockville, MD: National Institute on Drug Use.

Vigil, J. D. (1988). *Street Socialization, Locura Behavior, and Violence Among Chicano Gang Members*. Paper presented at the Research Conference on Violence and Homicide in Hispanic Communities, U of California, Los Angeles.

Vigil, J. D. (2000). *Community Dynamics and the Rise of Street Gangs.* Paper presented at the Latinos and the 21st Century: Mapping a Research Strategy, The David Rockefeller Center for Latin American Studies, Harvard University.

Wagner, F. A., & Anthony, J. C. (2002). From First Drug Use to Drug Dependence: Developmental Periods of Risk for Dependence upon Marijuana, Cocaine, and Alcohol. *Neuropsychopharmacology, 26*(4), 479-488.

Waldorf, D. (1993). When the Crips Invaded San Francisco–Gang Migration. *Journal of Gang Research, 1,* 11-16.

Zapert, K., Snow, D. L., & Tebes, J. K. (2002). Patterns of Alcohol and Other Drug Use in Early Through Late Adolescence. *American Journal of Community Psychology, 30*(6), 835-853.

Chapter 6

# Incarcerated Latinas and Alcohol and Other Drug Abuse: Assessment and Intervention Considerations

Betty Garcia, PhD

**SUMMARY.** An increase in incarceration rates and incidence of drug-related incarcerations for women has shown particularly high rates for ethnic women. Profiles of incarcerated women in general show a number of factors that create psychosocial obstacles. Recent statistics indicate that Latino women are twice as likely to be in prison in comparison to white female prisoners. The literature on Latinas and alcoholism and other drug abuse is reviewed, clinical observations of incarcerated Latinas are discussed and recommendations are presented for service delivery needs. *[Article copies available for a fee from The Haworth Document Delivery Service: 1-800-HAWORTH. E-mail address: <docdelivery@haworthpress.com> Website: <http://www.HaworthPress.com> © 2005 by The Haworth Press, Inc. All rights reserved.]*

**KEYWORDS.** Incarcerated Latinas, alcoholism and other drug abuse, diversity

Betty Garcia is Professor of Social Work, California State University, Fresno, 5310 N. Campus Drive, Fresno, CA 93740 (E-mail: bettyg@csufresno.edu).

[Haworth co-indexing entry note]: "Incarcerated Latinas and Alcohol and Other Drug Abuse: Assessment and Intervention Considerations." Garcia, Betty. Co-published simultaneously in *Alcoholism Treatment Quarterly* (The Haworth Press, Inc.) Vol. 23, No. 2/3, 2005, pp. 87-106; and: *Latinos and Alcohol Use/Abuse Revisited: Advances and Challenges for Prevention and Treatment Programs* (ed: Melvin Delgado) The Haworth Press, Inc., 2005, pp. 87-106. Single or multiple copies of this article are available for a fee from The Haworth Document Delivery Service [1-800-HAWORTH, 9:00 a.m. - 5:00 p.m. (EST). E-mail address: docdelivery@haworthpress.com].

doi:10.1300/J020v23n02_06

Recent decades have shown high incarceration and prison building rates in the U.S. (Dressel, 1994; Richie, 1996; Saari, 1987). California in particular allocates more funds towards prisons than towards higher education and has built twenty-one new prisons in the last 20 years compared to one public university campus (Butterfield, 1997). The increase of women in U.S. prisons has progressively grown in the last three decades. Between 1970 and 2001 female prison inmates increased from 5,635 to 85,031 (U.S. Department of Justice, 2001), and the growth between 1980 and 1992 represented a 225 percent increase compared to a 160 percent for men (Bureau of Justice Statistics, 1994b). The increase continued through the last decade of the 20th century with the female population increasing by 88% (Greenfeld & Snell, 1999). By 2002, women prisoners comprised 6.6% of all federal and state prisoners compared to 5.8% in 1993 (Bureau of Justice Statistics, 1994a; Harrison & Beck, 2002). Current statistics show a significant growth of women, drug involvement prior to incarceration and drug-related incarcerations (Greenfeld & Snell, 1999; Harrison & Beck, 2002).

This article will look specifically at incarcerated Latinas in relation to alcoholism and other drugs in general for the purpose of identifying population needs and service delivery implications. At-risk factors will be reviewed in order to provide a perspective within which to understand the specific drug use and dependence concerns encountered by incarcerated Latinas and recommendations for practice will be proposed. To begin, profile characteristics of incarcerated women in general, and Latino women in particular, and ecological concepts relevant for identifying needs and intervention implications for incarcerated Latinas will be addressed. The ecological concepts provide a framework that promotes identification of the assortment of factors that have a role in substance use such as culture, family system and access to services. Substance abuse findings will be discussed in relation to the findings relevant to incarcerated Latinas and will be supplemented by this writer's clinical practice observations in a prison setting. Special attention will be given to addressing the heterogeneity among Latino women inmates and its implications for practice. The term Latina will be used to refer to what is called Hispanic women, meaning females with national origins in Spanish language countries in the Americas. Also, the discussion is premised on recognition of remarkably influential characteristics such as national origin, immigration status, language dominance, acculturation, and discrimination that shape experience of Latinos (Manoleas & Garcia, 2003).

The profile of incarcerated women indicates that approximately 60% have histories of sexual or physical abuse, 37% have incomes of less than $600 per month, and about 30% receive social welfare assistance prior to their arrest (Greenfeld & Snell, 1999). Almost half have never married (Greenfeld & Snell, 1999) and approximately 65% and 59% of female state and federal prisoners, respectively, have minor children (Mumola, 2000). Between 1991 and 1999, the number of minor children with a parent in a prison increased from 936,500 to 1,498,800, with 22% of these children under the age of 5 years (Mumola, 2000). Latinas have been found (82%) to have minor children more often compared to African American (79.6%) or White (78.1%) incarcerated women (Snell & Morton, 1991).

The frequency of mental illness is higher for women in state prisons and local jails (25%) compared to men (16%) and twenty-two percent of Latino females in state prisons have been identified as mentally ill (Ditton, 1999). Between 42% to 55% of all mentally ill inmates reported a family member who has been incarcerated (Ditton, 1999). Snell and Morton (1991) found that 6.5% of incarcerated Latino women have "stayed overnight in a mental hospital or other mental health treatment center," and 12.1% had received prescription medication from a psychiatrist and another physician for emotional or mental problems since admission (p.10).

Ethnic women comprise 26.2% of the female population, and Latino women account for about 1 out of 7 women in state prisons and nearly 1 out of 3 in federal prisons (Greenfeld & Snell, 1999). Hispanic women have the lowest average age, 29.6, while White non-Hispanic women have the highest, 39.6 (Greenfeld & Snell, 1999). Moreover, between 1986 and 1996, the number of incarcerated Latino women increased from 11.7 to 14%, while in 1997 the Latino population comprised only 10.9% of the total population (www.census.gov/population/estimates/nation/intfile3-1.txt; www.census.gov/Press-Release/cb97-65.html), and they are almost twice as likely to be in prison as white female prisoners (Harrison & Beck, 2002; Snell & Morton, 1991).

The growth of women incarcerated for drug offenses reflects the war on crime strategy of mandatory minimum sentencing, which reduced the discretion of judges (Clear & Cole, 1994) in exercising flexibility in sentencing. Drug offenses account for 7% of growth among all Hispanic inmates between 1990 and 2000 (Harrison & Beck, 2002). However, there is also evidence of a rise in substance use among incarcerated females, as indicated in the finding that female inmates are five to eight times more likely to abuse alcohol, ten times more likely to abuse drugs and 27 times more likely to use cocaine compared to other women (Covington, 1998). Moreover, 62% and 37%, respectively, of women in state and federal prisons used drugs in the month before the offense, and 40% and 19%, respectively, in state and federal prisons were more likely to have committed their offense while under the influence of drugs (Mumola, 1999).

## ECOLOGICAL PERSPECTIVE IN FORENSIC SETTINGS

The ecological perspective view that behavior must be understood in relation to the systems with which a person interacts (Germain & Gitterman, 1999) is highly relevant for examining other drug abuse in Latinas and its implications for assessment and intervention. Ecological concepts emphasis on the role of a wide range of factors (e.g., personal, interpersonal, environmental), adaptive coping, and behavioral-environmental interrelatedness stimulates thoughtful assessment of factors that lead to problems in living (Germain, 1978; Meyer, 1988) and thus to substance use and abuse.

The ecological approach has specific helpful implications for addressing alcoholism and other drug concerns. For one, the multilevel perspective of practice suggests the necessity for sound skills needed to assess and intervene on an individual, family, group, organizational and policy level. Second, it acknowledges that practitioners providing alcoholism and other drug abuse services in correctional and community settings must deal with value differences related to diverse professional goals and strategies that impact the effectiveness of service delivery. Also, the court-involved nature of the client's situation that establishes the court as the client requires that service delivery practitioners work within the limitations imposed by the court (i.e., incarceration, parole status).

Third, the person environment interaction perspective promotes alcohol and other drug assessment to include a wide range of contextual factors such as family system, social support and psychological factors, social history and culture that can promote substance use (Amodeo & Jones, 1997, 1998; McNeece & DiNitto, 1998). Behavioral factors such as quantities, type and frequency of drugs, severity of drug use, patterns of use and experiences in abstinence (Connors, Donovan & DiClemente, 2001) can be evaluated in relation to supports and obstacles associated with sociocultural factors.

A person environment approach to alcoholism and other drug abuse promotes viewing health within a holistic rather than a fragmented manner. Ecological concepts emphasis on the interaction of various forces within an individual's life highlights the effects of stressors, coping styles and cultural forces into understanding what is often perceived as "individual choice." World Health Organization (WHO) public health researchers propose that conceptualization of health status needs to be broadened to include the impact on a population by premature death and disability by risk factors such as alcohol, sanitation and unsafe sex (Murray & Lopez, 1996). The WHO focus on "burden of disease" and inclusion of risk factors into an overall estimation of health status sharpens the focus on the complex nature of health and the unique constellation of factors associated with different populations.

The person environment approach promotes the identification of issues that are associated with alcoholism and other drug abuse that could exacerbate abuse and/or interfere with accessing services. For example, chemically dependent incarcerated women have been found to have higher rates of physical and/or sexual abuse histories and most often live at or below poverty levels (Austin, Bloom & Donahue, 1992). Incarcerated women are at risk for HPV (human papillomavirus) infection, HIV status, and other sexually transmitted diseases such as gonorrhea, syphilis and cervical dysplasia (Acoca, 1998; Bickell, Vermund, Holmes, Safyer & Burk, 1991; El-Bassell, Ivanoff, Schilling, Gilbert, Borne & Chen, 1995; Viadro & Earp, 1991). Hispanic women are at greater risk for HIV status, and are possibly three times more vulnerable, compared to White or African American women (Centers for Disease Control, 2000; Selik, Castro & Papaionnou, 1988; Snell & Morton, 1991). There is some evidence that Latinas are at risk for gallbladder problems, diabetes, tuberculosis, breast, cervical and colon cancer, heart disease cancer, and have a five times higher rate of primary and secondary syphilis than are White or African American women (Centers for Disease Control, 1993; Desenclos & Hahn, 1992; Frank-Stromberg, 1991; Flack, Amaro, Jenkins, Kunitz, Levy, Mixon & Yu, 1995; Haffner, Diehl, Mitchell, Stern & Hazuda, 1990; U.S. Dept. of Health & Human Services, 1986; Valdez, Delgado, Cervantes & Bowler, 1993; Zambrana & Ellis, 1995).

## *LATINAS: ALCOHOLISM AND OTHER DRUGS*

The 2000 census showed that Hispanics represent 12.5% of the population, with those of Mexican heritage representing 58.5% (Guzman,

2001). The large proportion of Mexican origin Latinos has led to substance use research primarily with this group. However, the discussion here builds from existing findings on alcoholism with this group and assessment considerations as a point of reference for examining ADOA issues with incarcerated Latinas of diverse national origins.

Mixed findings exist regarding whether Latino women consume less than Latino males (Caetano, Clark & Tam, 1998) or a higher prevalence of alcohol than Latino males (Xuequi & Shive, 2000). Time in the U.S., acculturation, divorced or single status, having some higher education, and a high income appear to constitute strong predictors of heavy alcohol use among Mexican American women (Black & Markides, 1993; Caetano, Clark & Tam, 1998; Caetano & Mora-Medina, 1988; Caetano, 1994; Canino, Burnam & Caetano, 1992; Gilbert & Collins, 1997). Mexican American women are more likely than immigrants to report parents with behavioral risk factors and women appear to be more susceptible to the effect of parent risk factors in the context of social and cultural assimilation (Rogler, Cortes & Malgady, 1991; Vega & Sribney, 2003). These findings are supported by findings on low levels of alcohol consumption found among recently immigrated Mexican women (Gilbert & Collins, 1997).

The little research that has been done on other substances indicates that Mexican American women have a higher prevalence of cocaine use compared to other Latino women (SAMHSA, 1993), and Mexican origin Latinos who spoke English were 25 times more likely to use cocaine (Amaro, Whitaker, Coffman & Heeren, 1990). Alvarez and Ruiz (2001) suggest that although Mexican Americans were found to have a higher use of illicit drug, methodological factors make it difficult to ascertain an accurate estimate. While alcoholism and other drug abuse data on Cuban women are lacking (Alvarez & Ruiz, 2001), there is some indication that Puerto Rican women have a higher lifetime use of cocaine than other Latino women and a high rate of heavy drinking (Alcocer, 1993; Alvarez & Ruiz, 2001; Booth, Castro & Anglin, 1990).

Research on alcoholism in women have identified patterns and themes that create several at-risk considerations. There is evidence that women with family histories of violence or alcoholism are at greater risk for alcoholism dependence (Chermack, Stoltenberg, Fuller & Blow, 2000) and are at greater risk for organ damage resulting from alcoholism than are men (van der Walde, Urgenson, Weltz & Hanna, 2002; Wilsnack, Wilsnack & Miller-Strumhofel, 1994). Also, alcoholism places the fetus at risk for numerous difficulties that include developmental delay, behavioral difficulties and fetal alcohol syndrome (West, Chen & Pantazis, 1994).

## INCARCERATED LATINAS

A few studies have focused specifically on the experiences and needs of incarcerated Latinas. Coll and Duff's (1995) study found that 83% were non-documented, 27.3% had left home before age 16, 75% did not have prior incarcerations, and 83% were convicted on a substance abuse-related crime. Although 45.5% reported alcohol use prior to incarceration, none reported daily use. Also, 58.3% and 50%, respectively, reported ongoing medical problems and significant critical life events twelve months prior to the incarceration (e.g., major illness, loss of a relationship) with 10% reporting the death of a child. Regarding future plans, 22.2% indicated they were concerned about coping with re-entry into the community and the adjustments needed for that transition. That 27.3% indicated that they did not feel that they had any skills, suggests many might not perceive themselves prepared to enter the job market upon release.

A subsample of 21 Latinas at a state prison (Garcia & Foster, 1997) indicated that Latina inmates had a mean age of 33.6, have a large representation of immigrants (n = 11), and the majority (n = 17) had minor children. Sixty-two percent described their health as good to poor, 71% indicated they felt their emotional or mental health was good to poor, and 43% indicated that they had received mental health treatment in the past five years for a wide range of problem areas that included post traumatic stress, affective and anxiety disorders.

Particularly relevant are Kail and Elberth's (2002) findings on Latina substance abusers that "gender and culture may serve to isolate the substance-abusing Latina, creating structural barriers to the identification of substance use as a problem" (p. 13). They propose that these two factors may be sufficiently powerful in supporting denial, such that directive, jolting strategies are needed that can nudge them into heeding the destructive consequences to themselves and their families (i.e., children). Examples of these prods include encounter with the justice system, removal of children, or reframing the problem as a serious medical concern. These researchers also point out the need for practitioners to explore the significance of working within a framework of traditional Latino beliefs, such as personalismo (i.e., interpersonal skill) and awareness of shame or stigma arising from seeking treatment information that may arise from gender role or culture.

Anecdotal data (Personal Communication, Rebecca Rodriguez, June 16, 2003) emerging from mental health practice in a prison substance abuse program identifies thought-provoking themes that bear scrutiny in evaluation and intervention planning activities. First, alcoholism and other drug abuse originating with family or significant others can have a powerful sway, particularly in a context of culturally based traditional gender role expectations that emphasize women's acquiescence. Second, alcohol abuse can be in addition to or secondary to illicit drug use of other more powerful substances. Assessment needs to review poly-substance abuse patterns of use and sociocultural factors that might have a role in maintaining use or impeding recognition and confrontation of addictive behavior. Third, variations in relation to factors that promote recovery may exist based on regional (e.g., northern or southern California) or national origin differences. Employability and possession of job skills are essential in providing a concrete foundation for empowerment, re-entering and becoming part of one's community. Without the prospect of future independence grounded in economic autonomy other options may be undermined and/or short-lived. These factors are essential to evaluate with the aim of promoting sufficient personal skills and resources in the lives of Latinas that will support them in their endeavors to manage the transition back into the community and so they may perhaps even flourish in their new efforts.

## INCARCERATED LATINAS: ASSESSMENT CONCERNS

The broad, inclusive approach to assessing alcohol and other drug abuse and its effects that is put forth here emphasizes the importance of attending to at-risk factors confronted by incarcerated Latinas based on their gender and ethnicity, assimilation, and incarceration and socioeconomic status (Deal & Galaver, 1994; Galea & Vlahov, 2002; Vega & Sribney, 2003). These factors include higher rates of mental disorders, suicidality, trauma experiences, substance abuse, reproductive health issues, violent victimization, HIV, infectious and communicable disease, diabetes, heart conditions and hypertension (Acoca, 1998; Carr, Hinkle & Ingram, 1991; Jordon, Schlenger, Fairbank & Caddell, 1996; Resnick, Kilpatrick, Dansky, Saunders & Best, 1993; Scott, Hannuum & Gilchrist, 1982; Singer, Bussey, Song & Lunghofer, 1995).

With almost one-third (30.3%) of Latinos living below the poverty level (www.census.gov/Press-Release/cb96-159a.html), socioeconomic status alone introduces vulnerability to distinct risks. Factors such as chronic life stressors, poverty, undereducation, underemployment and lack of access to adequate health services can disrupt the development of important resources such as social support and an independent, self-determined life (Zambrana & Ellis, 1995).

McNeece and DiNitto (1998) point out that assessment of ADOA addresses screening and diagnosis that deal with ascertaining abuse or dependency and confirmation of addictive difficulties. Assessment must be sufficiently comprehensive to assess polysubstance use and cover significant areas that include individual factors (e.g., education, employment, and military, medical, substance use, psychiatric and family history). It also needs to include information on court involvement, relationships with family members and why the client seeks help. Cultural factors need to be explored along with biological factors (Blume, 1998; Erickson & Wilcox, 2001) regarding such considerations as attitudes, values and behaviors related to using substances, and cultural factors related to acknowledging substance use as a problem, seeking help, relapse and maintaining recovery (Amodeo & Jones, 1998). In addition, an effective diversity-oriented perspective to assessment focuses on the significant factors such as socioeconomic class, religion or spirituality, age, rural or urban, resettlement, level of acculturation, context of immigration, and trauma (Amodeo & Jones, 1997).

## INCLUSIVE ASSESSMENT OF INCARCERATED LATINAS

The ecological approach and WHO "burden of disease" concept promote alcoholism and other drug abuse assessment of incarcerated Latinas and address the range of behavioral, social, cultural and environmental at-risk health factors confronted by Latinas dealing with alcoholism and other drugs. These perspectives promote assessment of essential domains such as history of physical and mental health treatment, undocumented status, cultural beliefs, values and attitudes about substance use and treatment, level of acculturation, family disengagement or cutoffs, alcoholism and other drug abuse and/or incarceration histories of the individual and the family. Furthermore, the profile also compels exploration of parenting role expectations, conflicts and stressors due to the high number with minor children.

Clinical observation and anecdotal data reveal stressors inherent in the incarceration experience related to unique psychosocial factors related to culture, socioeconomic status and social identity that bear attention in assessment and intervention planning. These include:

## Culture

Individual, cultural and organizational factors can contribute to barriers in women accessing needed prison-based health and psychological services, and in accessing community-based staff regarding their children's status and well-being. Language barriers can obstruct utilization of services needed for going into recovery as well as in establishing health practices vital to long-term well-being.

## Socioeconomic Status

At-risk factors associated with low income status contribute to greater prospects to lack of medical attention to health conditions that then have the potential of becoming chronic or life threatening, as with HIV status. Also, losses resulting from health problems or death of family members or vandalism of the inmate's community belongings are difficult for any individual, however, are worsened in a context of imprisonment.

## Isolation Within the Correctional Setting

The sense of isolation within the correctional setting, due to language and cultural differences, may provoke a lack of trust in prison physical and mental health services. These perceptions can lead to a lack of compliance with services and require active and extensive outreach efforts by prison staff and well developed human services programs. What may be perceived by staff as resistance may actually represent best efforts by the inmates at coping, based on perceptions from prior experience.

## Stressors Associated with Incarceration

Connections among incarcerated Latinas can be a double-edged sword. Nurturing supportive relationships among inmates can mediate the effects of alienation and isolation within the prison setting; however, clinical experience has shown that bearing witness to the painful adjustments of other Latinas and taking on a caregiving role can become a source of emotional pain that matches the pain with which the Latina, herself, is confronting. Although support from other Latinas is extremely valuable, this tie may also be the basis of an intensified sense of vulnerability. Clinical observations have also uncovered occasional instances where Latinas, in their cells, report to officers that they do not wish to attend group. However, immediate follow-up at the cell reveals that the prisoners in fact were too overwhelmed at that moment to participate in group and preferred an individual session.

## Program, Organizational, and Institutional Factors

Earnest attention needs to go to the assumptions underlying service delivery regarding practitioner awareness of consequences resulting from assumptions about alcoholism and "best practices" (i.e., as a disease or moral shortcoming). Ethnic and incarceration status and substance abusing difficulties can combine to evoke negative stereotypes from professionals that challenges them to uncover and work with the incarcerated woman's strengths.

Distance from the family and children posed by the location of the prison and language barriers in securing prison policy information that regulates visits can thwart and/or overshadow family visitations. Clear information regarding prison protocols regarding regulations such as acceptable visitor apparel (e.g., no blue clothing, even on infants and children) or quotas on the number of children who can visit in a day is essential. Family reliance on public transportation and coordination of documents for visitations can present cumbersome hurdles to manage for family visits.

## Family System

Clinical observations showed that many incarcerated Latinas had family histories characterized by disengagement and cutoffs as early as adolescence. Although some family contact may be tension producing, efforts should be expended to facilitate ongoing contact with natural support systems because of their potential for representing protective factors such as extended family, folk healers, religious affiliation, and social clubs (Delgado & Humm-Delgado, 1982).

The above considerations address the broad considerations necessary to bear in mind in practice with incarcerated Latinas and ADOA. The combination of research and anecdotal data arising from practice observations, however, reveal that substantive data on this population is hugely missing. We know little about the individual, family or alcoholism and other drug abuse patterns that lead to the incarceration of Latinas, particularly in relation to the heterogeneity within the group and how national origin and regional differences shape outcomes. The lack of data have implications for practice, in direct services and policy formation, as well as the development of a knowledge base grounded in research. The following recommendations are proposed in these areas.

## RECOMMENDATIONS

*Assessment.* Effective assessment requires particular consideration to polysubstance use, culture, family history, level of acculturation and is attuned to physical and mental health concerns related to population profile at-risk factors. A multisystem perspective gives due attention to individual, interpersonal and environmental factors, promotes identification of individual factors, such as poor judgment, as well as social forces related to socioeconomic limitations, gender role, cultural or family system dynamics. Patterns of polysubstance abuse need to be identified so that change efforts are premised on addressing the varieties of drug use. Identification of alcoholism and other drug abuse and examination of the origins of the behavior assist in maintaining recovery.

Family systems information is invaluable, particularly in instances where, as clinical observation has suggested, the Latina's alcoholism and other drug abuse is significantly influenced by intergenerational family substance abuse or pressures that evolve from intimate relationships with significant others and/or spouses. Such situations indicate equal attention in interventions to personal addictive behaviors and to interpersonal boundary issues.

*Culturally Competent Staffing and Intervention.* Culturally competent practice requires Spanish language fluency with monolingual Spanish speakers and even more important, culturally attuned interactions necessary for the most important skill of engagement. Engagement skills of practitioners are as significant as having knowledge of diverse cultures and awareness of the consequences of being culturally different. In addition, self-awareness of biases and negative stereotypes of incarcerated, Latino women with alcoholism and other drug problems have an important role as a focus in supervision. Pitfalls in practice include romanticizing the culture (i.e., seeing strength, where it is not) or overdiagnosis (i.e., seeing pathology where it is not). For example, in my clinical experience, a Latina inmate with an ataque de nervios precipitated by a major family loss was initially perceived by mental health staff as presenting psychotic behavior; however, she was correctly assessed as coping with an intense grieving process once staff communicated with the inmate in Spanish.

Questions of who can help whom in a context of diversity are best contemplated in relation to professional ethical behavior and the expectations of engaging with clients in a respectful fashion. All too often the daunting task of learning about others different from self can be inhibited by prematurely concluding professional ineffectiveness rather than engaging in the learning associated with developing new skills. The unique alcohol and other drug abuse issues and themes that arise in the lives of incarcerated Latinas must be dealt with as legitimate concerns that deserve exploration, clarification and integration into intervention goals.

*Continuity of Care.* Provision of health services must be comprehensive inside the prison and continue once the former inmate has returned to the community. The work in confronting the addiction, going into recovery and coping with relapse requires direction and support that needs to be grounded in continuity of care (Deitch, Carleton, Koutsenok & Marsolais, 2002). Service delivery should include individual, group and psychoeducational services, and in keeping with research findings, explore reframing the alcohol and other drug abuse problem for the purpose of heightening inmates' awareness of the damaging consequences of substance abuse.

Provision of alcohol and other drug abuse services inside and outside the correctional setting place tremendous importance on coordination and collaboration between prison and community-based services, both on inter-professional and inter-organizational levels. Collaboration builds shared responsibility taking. Such efforts between diverse professionals in corrections, medicine, and human services requires attunement and discussion about differences in professional ethics, values and practice approaches to alcohol and other drug abuse treatment. Social work professional values and concepts emphasize the recognition of multisystem factors that have a role in alcohol and other drug abuse such as gender role, culture and family system as well as a wide range of intervention strategies that include direct services, brokering and advocacy. Also, effective continuity of care between professionals involves professionals negotiating with other professions about the aims and significance of identified interventions.

There are several areas that should remain in focus for services in the prison and in the community. Building basic social skills necessary to maintain connections with others who support the Latinas' new goals and attending to the psychological and social consequences of the addictive behavior are priorities. Pre-release planning should include evaluation of the availability and/or development of social support for the purpose of planning for future stressors and options for coping. Depending on the inmate's desire to reunite with her children, staff can provide much needed assistance in maintaining communication with the children, caretakers and the children's protective services practitioners who may be involved.

*Appraising Assumptions in Service Delivery.* Several alternatives to the disease model (Jellinek, 1960) as a basis of treatment have come to the fore in recent years that expand the options for providing effective intervention goals and strategies that address the unique needs of incarcerated Latinas. For one, the harm reduction approach has gained recognition as a public health approach to intervention that provides a viable alternative to the corrections emphasis on demand reduction and criminalization of drug use rather than treatment (McNeece, 2003; McNeece, Bullington, Arnold & Springer 2001; Marlatt, 1998). As a "set of programs that share certain public health goals and assumptions" with the aim of changing substance abusing behavior towards the goal of minimizing the negative consequences (MacCoun, 1998), its outreach focus opens new possibilities for engaging individuals as well as communities in reducing substance abuse. Also, the stages of change model (Prochaska & DiClemente, 1992; DiClemente & Prochaska, 1998) that builds on the concept of identification of maladaptive behaviors for the purpose of change (Rinaldi, Steindler, Wilford & Goodwin, 1988) focuses on matching an individual's treatment to their commitment to change (Connors, Donovan & DiClemente, 2001) and offers a strength-based, process-oriented model. The stages of change model emphasis on attitudes, intentions and behaviors presents a concrete focus with which to identify the Latinas' limitations, values and strengths that can be explored in relation to their origins, and her needs, wants and hopes.

*Psychoeducational Interventions.* Several concerns that Latinas must struggle with can be addressed through psychoeducational resources to provide support for her behavioral change. These include: (1) The high percentage of incarcerated Latinas who have minor children suggests information and discussion on the biological effects of alcohol and other drugs on the female user and on a fetus can highlight the long-term and damaging risks involved. Likewise content on related issues such as domestic violence and the developmental effects on children can draw attention to the decisions that are being made and possible options. (2) The at-risk status of Latinas involved in substance abuse for HIV status and potentially for sexually transmitted diseases (STD) indicates a strong need for education and interventions directed at assisting

Latinas who have been diagnosed with either of these, as well as those who have not. The strong cultural inhibitions against dealing directly with these problems requires special consideration in addressing denial and shame that many Latinas may feel.

*Future Research.* The remarkable lack of empirical work on this population must be addressed with particular attention to polysubstance abuse. Research must target the content, dynamics and extent of polysubstance abuse for the purpose of identifying effective treatments (Alvarez & Ruiz, 2001) for the individual and family, and also direct prevention work in the community, as suggested by the harm reduction approach. Also, as research and clinical observations have shown, greater understanding is needed of the role of culture (Galaif & Newcomb, 1999), gender, family system and socioeconomic forces in initiating substance abuse, promoting polysubstance abuse, in obstructing recognition of an abuse problem and seeking assistance.

More information is essential on the heterogeneity and needs among Latinas on the basis of national origin, acculturation, socioeconomic and regional differences. Most of the research on alcoholism on Latinas is on Mexican Americans, with some comparisons between immigrant and middle income groups, with virtually no data on Latina populations in correctional settings. Data on family systems configurations, intergenerational alcohol and other drug abuse patterns and their effects on the female at different ages, experiences in coming to terms with the problem and seeking help are greatly needed to guide interventions within the prison and in community-based treatment. Incarcerated Latinas with substance abuse problems represent a highly marginalized population that receives little attention in the public eye and is usually presented in ways that promote negative stereotyping by providing scant information on the realities this highly diversified population confronts.

The significantly escalating numbers going into correctional settings and the increase in drug-related arrests accentuates the necessity of making this population and their needs more visible. The future of these women affects the well-being of their children and families, but also the health of the communities in which they live. Evidence shows that the constellation of factors that have a role and contribute to alcoholism and other substance abuse are varied and complex. This clearly calls for concerted efforts at all levels such as direct services, family intervention, policy formation and research to build a competent knowledge base for these efforts.

# REFERENCES

Acoca, L. (1998). Defusing the time bomb: Understanding and meeting the growing health care needs of incarcerated women. *Crime and Delinquency, 44*(1), 49-69.

Alcocer, A.M. (1993). Patterns of alcohol use among Hispanics. In R.S. Mayers, B.L. Kail & T.D. Watts (Eds.), *Hispanic substance abuse* (pp. 37-49). Springfield, IL: Thomas.

Alvarez, L.R. & Ruiz, P. (2001). Substance abuse in the Mexican population. In S.L.A. Straussner (Ed.), *Ethnocultural factors in substance abuse treatment.* New York: The Guilford Press.

Amaro, H., Whitaker, R., Coffman, G. & Heeren, T. (1990). Acculturation and marijuana and cocaine use: Findings from HHANES 1982-84. *American Journal of Public Health, 80* (Suppl.), 54-60.

Amodeo, M. & Jones, L.K. (1997). Viewing alcohol and other drug use cross culturally. *Families in Society, 78*(3), 240-254.

Amodeo, M. & Jones, L.K. (1998). Using the AOD cultural framework to view alcohol and drug issues through various cultural lens. *Journal of Social Work Education, 34*(3), 387-399.

Austin, J., Bloom, B. & Donahue, T. (1992). *Female offenders in the community: An analysis of innovative strategies and programs.* National Council on Crime and Delinquency. Washington, D.C.: National Institute of Corrections.

Bickell, N.A., Vermund, S., Holmes, M., Safyer, S. & Burk, R.D. (1991). Human papillomavirus, gonorrhea, syphilis, and cervical dysplasia in jailed women. *American Journal of Public Health, 81*(10), 1318-1320.

Black, S.A. & Markides, K.S. (1993). Acculturation and alcohol consumption in Puerto Rican, Cuban-American and Mexican American women in the United States. *American Journal of Public Health, 83*(6), 890-893.

Blume, S.B. (1998). Addiction in women. In *Textbook for substance-abuse treatment.* (2nd ed.) (pp. 485-490). Washington, D.C., American Psychiatric Press.

Booth, M.W., Castro, F.G. & Anglin, M.D. (1990). What do we know about Hispanic substance abuse? A review of the literature. In R. Glick & J. Moore (Eds.), *Drugs in Hispanic communities* (pp. 21-43). New Brunswick, NJ: Rutgers University Press.

Bureau of Justice Statistics. (1994a). *Bulletin: Prisoners in 1993.* Washington, DC: U.S. Government Printing Office.

Bureau of Justice Statistics. (1994b). *Special Report: Women in Prison.* Washington, DC: U.S. Government Printing Office.

Butterfield, F. (1997, September 28). Crime keeps on falling, but prisons keep on filling. *New York Times*, pp. 4-1, 4-4.

Caetano, R. (1994). Drinking and alcohol related problems among minority women. *Alcohol Health and Research World, 18*(3), 233-241.

Caetano, R. & Medina-Mora, M.E. (1988). Acculturation and drinking among people of Mexican descent in Mexico and the United States. *Journal of Studies on Alcohol, 49*, 462-471.

Caetano, R., Clark, C.L. & Tam, T. (1998). Alcohol consumption among racial/ethnic minorities: Theory and research. *Alcohol Research and Health, 22*(4), 233-238.

Canino, G., Burnam, A. & Caetano, R. (1992). The prevalence of alcohol abuse and/or dependence in two Hispanic communities. In J. Helzer & G. Canino (Eds.), *Alcoholism in North America, Europe and Asia* (pp. 131-154). New York: Oxford University Press.

Carr, K., Hinkle, B. & Ingram, B. (1991). Establishing mental health and substance abuse services in jails. *Journal of Prison & Jail Health, 10*(2), 77-89.

Centers for Disease Control. (1993). Advance report of final mortality statistics, 1990. *Morbidity and Mortality Weekly Report, 41*, 7.

Centers for Disease Control and Prevention. (2000). Division of HIV/AIDS Prevention: Basic statistics. Atlanta, GA.: Department of Health and Human Services [cited 2001 March 25]. Available from URL: *http://www.cc.gov/hiv/stats.htm.*

Chermack, S.T., Stoltenberg, S.F., Fuller, B.E. & Blow, F.C. (2000). Gender differences in the development of substance-related problems: The impact of family history of alcoholism, family history of violence and childhood conduct problems. *Journal of Studies on Alcohol, 61*, 845-852.

Clear, T. & Cole, G.F. (1994). *American corrections.* Belmont, CA: Wadsworth.

Coll, C.G. & Duff, K.M. (1995). *Reframing the needs of women in prison: A relational and diversity perspective.* Final Report. Women in Prison Pilot Project. Wellesley, MA: The Stone Center for Developmental Services and Studies.

Connors, G.J., Donovan, D.M. & DiClemente, C.C. (2001). *Substance abuse treatment and the stages of change.* New York: The Guilford Press.

Covington, S. (1998). Women in prison. Approaches in the treatment of our most invisible population. In J. Harden & Hill, M. (Eds.), *Breaking the rules: Women in prison and feminist therapy* (pp. 141-153). New York: The Haworth Press, Inc.

Deal, S.A. & Galaver, J. (1994). Are women more susceptible than men to alcohol . . . *Alcohol, Health & Research World, 18*, 189-191.

Deitch, D.A., Carleton, S., Koutsenok, I.G. & Marsolais, K. (2002). Therapeutic community treatment in prisons. In C.G. Leukefeld, F. Tims & D. Farabee (Eds.), *Treatment of drug offenders: Policies and issues.* New York: Springer Publishing Company.

Delgado, J. & Humm-Delgado, D. (1982). Natural support systems: Source of strengths in Hispanic communities. *Social Work, 27*, 83-89.

Desenclos, J.A. & Hahn, R.A. (1992). Years of potential life lost before age 65, by race, Hispanic origin, and sex–United States, 1986-1988. *Morbidity and Mortality Weekly Report, 42*.

DiClemente, C.C. & Prochaska, J.O. (1998). Toward a comprehensive transtheoretical model of change: Stages of change and addictive behaviors. In W.R. Miller & N. Heather (Eds.), *Treating addictive behaviors* (2nd ed.) (pp. 33-24). New York: Plenum Press.

Ditton, P.M. (1999). *Mental health and treatment of inmates and probationers.* Bureau of Justice Statistics NCJ 174463. Washington, D.C.: U.S. Department of Justice.

Dressel, P.L. (1994) . . . And we keep on building prisons: Racism, poverty, and challenges to the welfare state. Paper presented at the meeting of the Council on Social Work Education, Atlanta, GA.

El-Bassel, N., Ivanoff, A., Schilling, R.F., Gilbert, L., Borne, D. & Chen, D. (1995). Preventing HIV/AIDS in drug-abusing incarcerated women through skills building and social support enhancement: Preliminary outcomes. *Social Work Research*, *19*(3), 131-141.

Erickson, C.K. & Wilcox, R.E. (2001). Neurobiological causes of addiction. *Journal of Social Work Practice in the Addictions*, *1*(3), 7-22.

Flack, J.M., Amaro, H., Jenkins, W., Kunitz, S., Levy, J., Mixon, M. & Yu, E. (1995). Panel I.: Epidemiology of minority health. *Health Psychology*, *14*(7), 592-600.

Frank-Stromberg, M. (1991). Changing demographics in the United States. *Cancer*, *67*, 772-778.

Galaif, E.R. & Newcomb, M.D. (1999). Predictors of polydrug use among four ethnic groups. *Addictive Behaviors*, *24*(5), 607-631.

Galea, S. & Vlahov, D. (2002). Social determinants and the health of drug users: Socioeconomic status, homeless, and incarceration. *Public Health Reports*, *117*(3), 135-145.

Garcia, B. & Foster, B. (1997). Incarcerated women and child welfare issues: A systems perspective on implications for practice. Unpublished raw data.

Germain, C. (1978). General-systems theory and ego psychology: An ecological perspective. *Social Service Review*, *52*(4), 535-550.

Germain, C.B. & Gitterman, A. (1999). Ecological perspective. In *Encyclopedia of social work* (19th ed.). Washington, D.C.: National Association of Social Workers.

Gilbert, M.J. & Collins, R.L. (1997). Ethnic variation in women's and men's drinking. In R.W. Wilsnack & S.C. Wilsnack (Eds.), *Gender and alcohol*. New Brunswick, NJ: Rutgers Center of Alcohol Studies, pp. 357-378.

Greenfeld, L.A. & Snell, T.L. (1999). *Women offenders*. NCJ 175688. Washington, D.C.: U.S. Department of Justice.

Guzman, B. (2001). *The Hispanic population: Census 2000 brief*. Washington, D.C.: U.S. Department of Commerce.

Haffner, S.M., Diehl, A.K., Mitchell, B.D., Stern, M.P. & Hazuda, H.P. (1990). Increased prevalence of clinical gallbladder disease in subjects with non-insulin-dependent diabetes mellitus. *American Journal of Epidemiology*, *132*(2), 327-335.

Harrison, P.M. & Beck, A.J. (2002). Prisoners in 2001. *Bureau of Justice Statistics Bulletin*. NCJ 195189. Washington, D.C.: U.S. Department of Justice.

Jellinek, E. (1960). *The disease concept of alcoholism*. New Haven, CT: College and University Press.

Jordan, B.K., Schlenger, W.E., Fairbank. J.A. & Caddell, J.M. (1996). Prevalence of psychiatric disorders among incarcerated women. *Archives of General Psychiatry*, *53*(6), 513-519.

Kail, B.L. & Elberth, M. (2002). Moving the Latina substance abuser toward treatment: The role of gender and culture. *Journal of Ethnicity in Substance Abuse*, *1*(3), 3-16.

MacCoun, R.J. (19998). Toward a psychology of harm reduction. *American Psychologist*, *3*(11), 1199-1208.

Manoleas, P. & Garcia, B. (2003). Clinical algorithms as a tool for psychotherapy with Latino clients. *American Journal of Orthopsychiatry*, *73*(2), 154-166.

Marlatt, G.A. (1998). Basic principles and strategies of harm reduction. In G.A. Marlatt (Ed.), *Harm reduction* (pp. 49-68). New York: The Guilford Press.

McNeece, C.A. (2003). After the war on drugs is over: Implications for social work education. *Journal of Social Work Education*, *39*(2), 193-212.

McNeece, C.A., Bullington, B., Arnold, E.M. & Springer, D.W. (2001). The war on drugs. In R. Muraskin & A.R. Roberts, *Visions for change: Crime and justice in the twenty-first century* (3rd ed.). Upper Saddle River, N.J.: Prentice Hall.

McNeece, C.A. & DiNitto, D.M. (1998). *Chemical dependency: A systems approach* (2nd ed.). Boston: Allyn and Bacon.

Meyer, C. (1988). The eco-systems perspective. In R.A. In Dorfman (Ed.), *Paradigms of clinical social work*. New York: Brunner/Mazel.

Mumola, C.J. (1999). Substance abuse and treatment, state and federal prisoners, 1997. *Bureau of Justice Statistics Special Report*. Washington, D.C.: U.S. Department of Justice.

Mumola, C.J. (2000). Incarcerated parents and their children. Bureau of Justice Statistics, NCJ 182335. Washington, D.C.: U.S. Department of Justice.

Murray, C. & Lopez, A.D. (1996). *The global burden of disease*. Cambridge, MA: The Harvard School of Public Health.

Proschaska, J.O. & DiClemente, C.C. (1992). Stages of change in the modification of problem behaviors. In M. Hersen, R.M. Eisler & P.M. Miller (Eds.), *Progress in behavior modification*. Vol. 28 (pp. 183-218).

Resnick, H.S., Kilpatrick, D.G., Dansky, B.S., Saunders, B.E. & Best, C.L. (1993). Prevalence of civilian trauma and posttraumatic stress disorder in a representative national sample of women. *Journal of Consulting Clinical Psychology, 61*, 984.

Richie, B.E. (1996). *Compelled to crime*. New York: Routledge.

Rinaldi, R.C., Steindler, E.M., Wilford, B.B. & Goodwin, D. (1988). Clarification and standardization of substance abuse terminology. *Journal of American Medical Association, 259*, 555-557.

Rogler, L.H., Cortes, D.E. & Malgady, R.B. (1991). Acculturation and mental health status among Hispanics. *American Psychologist, 46*(6), 585-597.

Sametz, L. (1980). Children of incarcerated women. *Social Work, 25*(4), 298-303.

Saari, R.C. (1987). The female offender and the criminal justice system. In D.S. Burden & N. Gottlieb (Eds.), *The woman client*. New York: Tavistock Publications.

Scott, N.A., Hannum, T.E. & Chilchrist, S.L. (1982). Assessment of depression among incarcerated females. *Journal of Personality Assessment 46*, 372-379.

Selik, R., Castro, K. & Papaionnou, M. (1988). Racial/ethnic differences in the risk of AIDS in the U.S. *American Journal of Public Health, 78*, 1539-1544.

Singer, M.I., Bussey, J., Song, L. & Lunghofer, L. (1995). The psychosocial issues of women serving time in jail. *Social Work, 40*(1), 103-113.

Snell, T.L. & Morton, D.C. (1991). *Women in prison*. Washington, D.C.: Bureau of Justice Statistics, Special Report.

Stephan, J. & Jankowski, L. (1991). *Jail inmates, 1990*. Washington, D.C.: Department of Justice.

Substance Abuse and Mental Health Services Administration. (1993). *1991-1993 National household survey on drug abuse*. Washington, DC: U.S. Government Printing Office.

U.S. Department of Health and Human Services. (1986). *Report of the Secretary's task force on Black and minority health: Vol. VIII. Hispanic health issues*. Washington, DC: U.S. Government Printing Office.

U.S. Department of Justice. (1991). *Women in prison*. Washington, D.C.: U.S. Government Printing Office.

U.S. Department of Justice. (2001). Bulletin. NCJ 195189, p. 6. Washington, D.C.: Author.

Valdez, R.B., Delgado, D.J., Cervantes, R.C. & Bowler, S. (1993). *Cancer in U.S. Latino communities: An exploratory review*. Santa Monica, CA: Rand.

van der Walde, H., Urgenson, F., Weltz, S. & Hanna, F. (2002). Women and alcoholism: A biopsychosocial perspective and treatment approach. *Journal of Counseling and Development, 80*(2), 145-153.

Vega, W.A. & Sribney, W. (2003). Parental risk factors and social assimilation in alcohol dependence of Mexican Americans. *Journal of Studies on Alcohol, 64*(2), 167-175.

Viadro, C.I. & Earp, J.A. (1991). AIDS education and incarcerated women: A neglected opportunity. *Women and Health, 17*(2), 105-117.

West, J.R., Chen, W.A. & Pantazis, N.J. (1994). Fetal alcohol syndrome: The vulnerability of the developing brain and possible mechanisms of damage. *Metabolic Brain Disease, 9*(29), 291-322.

Wilsnack, R.W., Wilsnack. S.C. & Miller-Strumhofel, S. (1994). How women drink: Epidemiology of women's drinking and problem drinking. *Alcohol Health and Research World, 18*, 173-181.

Xuequi, G. & Shive, S. (2000). A comparative analysis of perceived risks and substance abuse among ethnic groups. *Addictive Behaviors, 25*(3), 361-371.

Zambrana, R.E. & Ellis, B.K. (1995). Contemporary research issues in Hispanic/Latino women's health. In D. Adams (Ed.), *Health issues for women of color*. Thousand Oaks, CA: Sage Publications.

Chapter 7

# Ahora le Voy a Cuidar Mis Nietos: Rural Latino Grandparents Raising Grandchildren of Alcohol and Other Drug Abusing Parents

## Karen Bullock, PhD

**SUMMARY.** The abuse of alcohol and other substances has long been the source of disruption in family structures and lifestyles. Yet, the impact on Latino grandparent-headed households in rural communities has received little attention to date. Health and social services agencies can reach out to rural elderly Latinos by involving community representatives in the intervention process and making culturally sound recommendation for practice and program development. *[Article copies available for a fee from The Haworth Document Delivery Service: 1-800-HAWORTH. E-mail address: <docdelivery@haworthpress.com> Website: <http://www.HaworthPress.com> © 2005 by The Haworth Press, Inc. All rights reserved.]*

**KEYWORDS.** Elderly Latinos, grandparents raising grandchildren

Karen Bullock is Assistant Professor of Social Work, University of Connecticut School of Social Work, 1798 Asylum Ave., West Hartford, CT 06117-2698.

[Haworth co-indexing entry note]: "Ahora le Voy a Cuidar Mis Nietos: Rural Latino Grandparents Raising Grandchildren of Alcohol and Other Drug Abusing Parents." Bullock, Karen. Co-published simultaneously in *Alcoholism Treatment Quarterly* (The Haworth Press, Inc.) Vol. 23, No. 2/3, 2005, pp. 107-130; and: *Latinos and Alcohol Use/Abuse Revisited: Advances and Challenges for Prevention and Treatment Programs* (ed: Melvin Delgado) The Haworth Press, Inc., 2005, pp. 107-130. Single or multiple copies of this article are available for a fee from The Haworth Document Delivery Service [1-800-HAWORTH, 9:00 a.m. - 5:00 p.m. (EST). E-mail address: docdelivery@haworthpress.com].

## INTRODUCTION

The abuse of alcohol and other substances has long been the source of disruption in family structures and lifestyles. The 1990s ushered in a new phenomenon for American society, which according to research (Anglin, 1990; Burnette, 1999b; Burton, 1992; Roe, Minkler, & Barnwell, 1994), has been influenced by the pervasiveness of drug problems among various ethnic groups. Grandparents as parents, in households where they provide primary care for a child in the absence, inability, or unwillingness of the parents (Karp, 1993), are increasing at an unprecedented rate (Casper & Bryson, 1998). The long history of research and practice efforts to curb the demonstrated relationship between substance use and a plethora of other social problems that often result in negative family crises (Anhalt & Klein, 1979; Jessor, 1976; Kandel & Logan, 1984; Marsigalia & Daley, 2002; National Institute on Drug Abuse, 1990; Napier, Bachtel, & Carter, 1983; Zambrana, 1987) has fallen short of averting the grandparent as parent (GAP) phenomena, where the child's parent is not present in the home. Although alcohol, drugs and other substances are frequently identified as critical factors in the neglect of children across cultures (De La Rosa, Segal, & Lopez, 1999; McMahon, Winkel, Suchman, & Luthar, 2002; Roe, Minkler, & Barnwell, 1994), the impact on Latino grandparent-headed households in rural communities has received little attention in the social science literature.

The present article seeks to add grandparenting to the alcohol and other drug abuse research agenda by describing the subjective perception of the impact that these drugs has on the grandparents as parents in a rural Latino community in the southeastern region of the United States (U.S.). Specific areas of inquiry were stressors, sacrifices, and service needs precipitated by substance-abusing parents of grandchildren who were in the primary care of grandparents. Several key assumptions are identified to guide practitioners in both assessing rural Latino grandparent-headed families and planning culturally appropriate intervention.

## BACKGROUND

It is well known that Latinos are the fastest growing population in the United States. What is less emphasized, however, is the rapid rate at which the growth is occurring in rural areas versus urban cities (U.S. Census, 2002) and the literature on grandparents raising grandchildren continues to overlook this group. Overall, there is a dearth of information about custodial grandparents of color, living in rural areas.

Although a growing body of data is available on needs and problems encountered by grandparents as parents (Cox, Brooks, & Valcarcel, 2000; Poindexter & Linsk, 1999; Pruchno & McKenney, 2002), including a decade of national surveys (Fuller-Thomson & Minkler, 2000), there are a number of important research questions that are yet to be addressed. This is due in part to the fact that the vast majority of the research has ignored those families living in rural, densely settled areas and this assessment applies even more critically to the current state of knowledge about impact of on Latino grandparents who parent in rural areas.

Despite the paucity of research on the impact of alcohol and other drug abuse on Latino grandparents in rural areas, much has been written to document the commonalities and differences among grandparents across ethnic groups. Studies have highlighted the self-reports of mostly grandmothers because women are more likely than men to assume the role of caregiver (Tennstedt, 1999) and take primary responsible for a grandchild's activities of daily living when co-residency occurs (Bullock, 2001).

## *Empirical Foundation for Understanding the "GAP" Phenomenon*

The role adjustment from grandparent to parent has reportedly brought on physical and emotional stress (Burnette, 1999c) as well as psychological (Kelley, Whitley, Sipe, & Yorker, 2000) and social service needs (Cox, 2002). In a qualitative study of 71 African American grandmothers caring for grandchildren of the crack-cocaine epidemic, these grandparents reported a lost of freedom and feelings of being cheated by the parent of the grandchild. At a time when many elders look ahead to retirement, these grandparents said they felt a sense of moving backward in life as they had to give up their job to parent at an "off time." Yet, many were able to identify positive attributes of the role of grandparent as parent (Roe, Minkler, & Barnwell, 1994).

In a largely white sample of grandparents as parents, another study found that grandparents who co-resided shared uncertainty and worry regarding their role as parent, along with concern about the level of family disruption that the grandchild could experience (Jendrek, 1994). When focusing on black grandparents, including grandfathers, and great-grandmothers as parents, Burton (1992) found that almost all (86%) reported their feelings of anxiety or depression as being directly related to parent stress; most (61%) reported increased health risk of smoking; while many (36%) reported increased alcohol consumption, and almost an equal number to those (35%) reported aggravated arthritis or diabetes.

Grandparents as parents make a range of sacrifices in order to raise grandchildren. They tend to minimize their own social (Jendrek, 1994) and health (Whitley, Kelley, & Sipe, 2001) needs. The time for relaxation and rest is often compromised as well as time to socialize with their adult peers (Musil, Youngblut, Ahn, & Curry, 2001). What is not clear from the research is whether grandparents feel they are making sacrifices in regards to their interaction or lack of interaction with the substance abusing parent. Given the potential impact of stress and sacrifices on grandparents as parent, there is a clear need to expand the body of knowledge available on relative risk factors associated with taking on the role of primary caregiver for a grandchild.

It is not clear whether service needs, as expressed by Latino grandparents, in rural areas differ from those in urban areas. But what is known about the needs of those who are raising their grandchildren in a vastly different time and cultural milieu from that which they raised their own children is that culturally specific educational, financial, and peer support services (Cox, Brooks, & Valcarcel, 2000) are a must.

## *Conceptual Foundations for Understanding Grandparents as Parent Phenomenon*

One of the most promising conceptual frameworks is social adaptation (Vega, 1990), a structural approach in which increased attention is paid to the social situations and contexts that affect Latino families. It has been argued, "the most pervasive problem of today's family life has to do with its felt loss of resources and the imminent threat of abandonment and fragmentation" (Boszormenyi-Nagy & Krasner, 1986, p. 57). Grandparents who assume the role of parent due to alcohol and other drug abuse issue of their offsprings are forced to deal with a range of stressors, sacrifices, service needs (Burton, 1992; Hirshorn, Meter, & Brown, 2000) each of which can be brought on by a loss of resources. One of the greatest losses of resources might be that of available parents to raise their children. The absent parent creates a "gap" in the family system and according to Soriano (1993) Latinos are disproportionately affected by the social problems of substance use and abuse. Nonetheless, older adults in rural areas, reportedly (Stoller, 1998), serve as symbols of family continuity and family crisis arbitrators. For the substance abusing parents in small densely settled communities, there may be less of a "gap" given that the rural context usually means living within close proximity of one another or at least in the same community. For grandparents in rural towns, their self-reliance, mutual support, and rurality may help to keep them isolated and underserved (Carlton-LaNey, 1992).

The distress parents experience when drug and alcohol abuse compromise their ability to care for their children, has been documented through both qualitative (Kearney, Murphy, & Rosenbaum, 1994) and quantitative (McMahon, Winkle, Suchman, & Luthar, 2002) studies. There is agreement that no time is a good time to be confronted with issues of alcohol and other drug abuse, but when grandparents find themselves, late in life, in the role of parent and managing the outcomes of abandonment, neglect, and abuse experienced by grandchildren (Whitley, Kelley, & Sipe, 2001), the "time-disordered roles" can be overwhelming. The assumption is these roles are enacted when an "individual's various social spheres and role sets are not temporally synchronized" (Seltzer, 1976, pp. 111-112).

Nonetheless, studies exploring substance abusing parents (Parke, 2002; Suchman & Luthar, 2000) suggest that compromise of parenting otherwise attributable to abuse of illicit and prescription drugs, including over the counter medications and alcohol (Gorman-Smith, Tolan, Henry, & Leventhal, 2002) may be mediated by a number of social, familial and individual factors. Conceptual links between alcohol and other drug abuse and grandparenting are important because there is accumulating evidence both within (Jendrek, 1994) and across cultures (Cox, Brooks, & Valcarcel, 2000; Gibson, 2002) that grandparents can have a positive impact on the adjustment of grandchildren for whom they provide primary care. Yet, they compromise their own economic security, health and social well-being.

The context in which many Latinos experience rural conditions provides some direction for locus of exploration. The growth of Latinos in the southeastern part of the U.S. has resulted primarily from the expanding opportunities for seasonal and permanent employment in agricultural production manufacturing, construction, and services positions. The population tends to be younger than retirement age (65 years) and mostly Mexicans who migrate from small villages in Mexico. A smaller percentage has spent some time in more urban areas prior to moving to the rural southeast (NC Office of Minority Health, 1999). The fact that the etiology of alcohol and other drug abuse among Latinos can be traced to uprooting, acculturation, and limited resources (Philleo & Brisbane, 1995) puts these families at risk. Consequently, to the extent that drug and alcohol abuse is leading to the unavailability of parents to care for their children, there is a need for more insight into the role of Latino grandparent as parent in a rural context. The relative absence of information about the influence of contextual factors within specific cultures is an important one to note. Burton (1992) suggests that contextual factors can greatly influence a grandparent's ability to perform "time disordered roles" such as parenting a grandchild.

## METHODS

### Sample

This sample of Latino grandparents, mostly Mexican, who participated in this study of the impact of alcohol and other drug abuse on grandparenting was drawn from a larger comparative observational study of African American, Latino, and white elders that looked at the changing role of grandparents raising grandchildren in a rural southeastern region. The grandparents were responsible for the primary care of at least one grandchild under the age of 18. For the larger study, recruitment for the research study was first introduced to the potential respondents either at a church event or some other community-based agency. In some cases, members of a social network provided the name and address of the grandparent so that recruitment could be facilitated through telephone calls and mailings. Grandparents responded to recruitment materials by contacting the project staff at a community agency via telephone or on a walk-in basis. At that point, participants were informed of the study requirements and screened for eligibility (grandparent as parent). Each Spanish-speaking participant was mailed an informed consent form and other study materials that included an introduction letter, which further explained the two-part interview process and a return-addressed stamped envelope to confirm receipt of study materials. For respondents with Spanish surnames and/or who identified a language preference at screening, all documents were in both English and Spanish. After the initial mailing, a reminder was sent to those who met the research eligibility requirements along with a survey questionnaire. The grandparents were given the option to complete the survey instrument prior to or at the same time as the in-person, qualitative interview. The sample was created by response rate.

Upon completing the interview process in its entirety, Latino families were asked to identify another Latino grandparent headed-household for potential participation in the study. This snowball technique, which has been validated in previous studies in Latino communities (Calderón & Tennstedt, 1998), was incorporated to increase the likelihood of locating grandparents in rural areas where it was thought that many were migrant farm workers (NC Office of Minority Health, 1999).

The respondents for the present study were older women (n = 50), ranging in age 60-84 years, all of whom identified substance use or abuse as factor in their assuming the role of parent. Table 1 shows the selected background characteristics of the respondents. Only grandmothers completed the interviews, although 20 percent of the families considered themselves to be two-grandparent households. Participation in the study was purely voluntary and no incentive was provided except transportation to and from the interview, when needed.

It was explained to the grandparents that the confidential data collected from them would be useful to professionals in identifying the specific needs of Spanish speakers in rural area. Language is believed to be the common characteristic that links the quite diverse U.S. population of Latinos (Toledo, Hayslip, Emick, Toledo, & Henderson, 2000). A large percentage of Latinos in the region where the data was collected speak only Spanish, with the others speaking mostly Spanish (NC Minority Health, 1999).

### Data Collection

Survey interviews were conducted in both English and Spanish, using back-translation techniques (Becerra & Shaw, 1988) for English to Spanish equivalents of the survey instruments. Only two interviews were completed in English by respondent preference. More than half of the interviews took place in a community agency (60%), while the others were completed in the living quarters, not necessarily that of the grandparent and not necessarily considered to be their homes, but temporary housing arrangement. The respondents interviewed in the agency were similar to those interviewed in a residence, except those interviewed in an agency were more likely to be married. Each respondent completed a questionnaire that consisted of a checklist as an interview guide, including the Parenting Stress Index/Short Form (PSI/SF, Abidin, 1995).

The qualitative component of the study consisted of an additional data collection process, which included face-to-face individual interviews, with open-ended questions. This allowed the grandparents to elaborate their concerns without having to fit them into predetermined constructs. This also enabled the research to be steeped in the meaning that these particular rural dweller give to their experiences. Interviews

TABLE 1. Latino Grandparent Participants (N = 50)

| Individual Variables: Selected Background Characteristic | Percent |
|---|---|
| *Gender* | |
| Female | 100 |
| | |
| *Age* | |
| 60-74 | 50 |
| 75-84 | _50_ |
| | 100 |
| *Health Status* | |
| Fair | 66 |
| Poor | 40 |
| Don't know | _4_ |
| | 100 |
| *Marital Status* | |
| Never married | 2 |
| Married/living w/spouse | 26 |
| Married/not living w/spouse | 20 |
| Separated/not living w/spouse | 15 |
| Widowed | 33 |
| Divorced | _4_ |
| | 100 |
| *Education* (highest graded completed) | |
| None | 10 |
| Some elementary school | 20 |
| Completed elementary school | 34 |
| Some middle school | 20 |
| Completed middle school | 6 |
| Some high school | _10_ |
| | 100 |
| *Years in the Continental U.S.* | |
| < 10 | 10 |
| 11-20 | 38 |
| 20+ | _52_ |
| | 100 |
| *Monthly Net Household Income* | |
| Under $600 | 64 |
| $600.00-$899.00 | 30 |
| $900.00+ | _6_ |
| | 100 |

were audio-taped, with written consent of the interviewees, and transcribed for coding and analysis.

## Variables

To better understand the stressors, sacrifices, and service needs of rural Latino grandparent-headed families, the survey instrument included demographic questions, which allow for the description of this population and their parenting arrangements due to alcohol and other drug abuse. Univariate (frequency distributions and mean) and bivariate (chi-square) statistics were used (see Table 1 for sample characteristics). To collect data on the individual level, following variables were considered in the analyses for grandparents: gender, age, health status (self-report), education (years of school completed), co-residency with spouse or partner, years in continental United States and income. The characteristics of the substance abusing parents as reported by the grandparents were included in order to assess the familial dynamics. They were as follows: the relationship to the grandparent, marital status, occupation, proximity to grandparent as parent (measured in distance) and drug of choice. Contextual characteristics of the caregiving situation were also considered. Those variables were number of children living in the grandparent-headed household, age of grandchild(ren) at the time of the interview, reasons for assuming and continuing in the parenting role, contact with the substance abusing parent (yes/no) and the rurality of their environment (farm town versus non-farm town).

Parenting stress was measured through the use of the Parenting Stress Index/Short Form (PSI/SF, Abidin, 1995). This instrument is designed to assess the degree to which stress exists in the parent-child system. However, the measure has been used in grandparent studies (Kelley, 1993). The index measured the overall level of parenting stress and factors in three subscales measuring specific domains of parenting stress: parenting distress, parent-child dysfunctional interaction, and perceptions of a difficult child. The subscales contained 12 items with a five-point scale rating, where higher scores indicated greater distress. The parenting distress subscale considered the grandparent's self-esteem, sense of competence, and role restriction. The parent-child dysfunctional interaction subscale evaluated the grandparent-grandchild bond and the degree to which the child met the grandparent's expectations. A sample question was "when I do things for my (grand) child, I get the feeling my efforts are not appreciated very much." The difficult child subscale appraised behavioral and temperamental characteristics of the child. The PSI has been used extensively in research studies and its validity has been confirmed through its utility with various populations including at-risk families.

## ANALYSIS

Data were entered and analyzed utilizing SPSS procedures. Pearson product moment correlations and step-wise multiple regression were conducted to examine relationships among study variables and dependent measures. Alpha reliability coefficients have been determined with a total score of .94, with subscales for each domain being .82 to .89. Test-retest reliability has been supported by various studies.

Grandparents were asked a series of open-ended questions about experiences and feelings that they may have about the impact of alcohol and other drug abuse on their assuming the role of parent for their grandchild. For this particular study, those narratives were used in these analyses. The individual interview data were analyzed through transcription of the taped interview sessions of personal accounts from the open-ended questions. Each of these data sources was analyzed in a paragraph-by-paragraph manner where each paragraph was assessed based on its content. Next each paragraph or related section was assigned a theme indicating the predominant theme is contained. Finally the themes themselves were analyzed in order to ferret out the common and most frequently occurring themes in the qualitative data.

## RESULTS

### Grandparents as Parents Due to Alcohol and Other Drug Abuse

The elderly Latino grandmothers who were parenting grandchildren due to problems of alcohol and other drug abuse in the family ranged from ages 60-84 years old. Forty-six percent of the respondents were married. Yet, the living arrangements for 20 percent of them were not consistent with this report, due to demands of migrant farm work that often meant the spouse worked away from the family for periods of time. More than half (54%) of the women reported that they were not living with their spouse or partner.

Generally, these women perceived their health as fair to poor (Table 1). Previous research has confirmed that migrant farm worker families tend not to be a healthy population (Alderete, Vega, Kolody, & Aguilar-Gaxiola, 2000). Most of the Latino elders completed elementary school (52%) but some did not (30%) and few completed high school (10%). The majority (66%) of the participants had extremely low (less than $600) monthly household incomes. The vast majority of these respondents had resided in the continental U.S. for less than 20 years (80%), with 20 percent having lived in the U.S. for a longer period of time.

## The Substance Abusing Parent

Sons were mostly likely to be the alcohol or other drug abusing parent. By and large, the women in these rural towns were paternal grandmothers (94%). This finding is consistent with the literature on comprised parenting by fathers in the Latino and American culture (Fox & Solis-Camara, 1997). Only 4 percent of the grandparents were maternal grandmothers caring for children of substance abusing women. Of these substance abusing men and women, 28 percent were identified as married and living with their spouses (Table 2). As has been the case with other rural populations (NC Office of Minority Health, 1999), all of these parents were reported to have had primary employment in agricultural, low-skill service jobs or were unemployed at the time of data collection. However, unlike reports on other rural populations (Carlton-LaNey, 1992; Stoller, 1998) these Latino parents were most often not living within close proximity of their families, with about half of grandparenting reporting in their narratives that they did not know the whereabouts of the substance abusing parent. This may have been related to the fact that migrant men tend to go back and forth between the U.S. and their native homelands when faced with stressors and crises (Purnell, 1998). With reported histories of drug and alcohol abuse, according to the grandparents, these parents most frequently used alcohol (100%) and marijuana (56%).

## Grandparenting in the Rural Context

All of the grandparents in this sample were living in farm towns. According to the literature (Stoller, 1998), rural farm towns have been in crisis since the 1980s, plagued by economic depression, layoffs from agricultural industries, increased poverty rates and farm foreclosures. With 65 percent of the grandparent-headed families adding one grandchild to their household and the remaining 35 percent parenting two grandchildren (see Table 3), the rural context has the potential to exacerbate the stress of managing the responsibilities. Of grandchildren in the care of these elderly grandparents, almost all (80%) of them were younger than school age (6 years) at the time of the interview. Each of the respondents reported alcohol or drugs as a factor that influenced their decision to assume parental care for their grandchild. When asked,

TABLE 2. Parental Alcohol and Other Drug Abusers

| Familial Variables: Selected Characteristics | Percent |
|---|---|
| *Relationship to the Grandparent as Parent* | |
| Son | 96 |
| Daughter | 4 |
| | 100 |
| | |
| *Marital Status* | |
| Never married | 20 |
| Married/living w/spouse | 28 |
| Married/not living w/spouse | 34 |
| Separated/not living w/spouse | 10 |
| Widowed | 2 |
| Divorced | 6 |
| | 100 |
| | |
| *Occupation* | |
| Mechanics | 20 |
| Crop harvest | 36 |
| Landscape | 24 |
| Day labor | 8 |
| Unemployed | 12 |
| | 100 |
| *Proximity to Grandparent as Parent* | |
| < 1 mile | 2 |
| > 1 but less than 20 miles | 16 |
| > 20 but less than 50 miles | 10 |
| > 50 but less than 100 | 20 |
| > 100 | 52 |
| | 100 |

"Please tell me how the alcohol and other drug abuse . . . led to your taking responsibility for the grandchild," neglect related to parental alcohol and other drug abuse (36%) was most often identified as the reason that the child was now in the grandparent care. Abandonment was sited in 24 percent of the cases, physical abuse of the child being reported 20 percent of the time, with other domestic violence being reported by 14 percent of the families and even fewer respondents reported fear of the alcohol and other drug abusers as the motive for taking the grandchild in. Over half of the grandparents had no contact with the alcohol and

TABLE 3

| Description of Context Variables (N = 50) | Percent |
| --- | --- |
| *Number of Grandchildren Living in the Home* | |
| One | 65 |
| Two | 35 |
| | 100 |
| | |
| *Current Age of Grandchild* | |
| < 1 year-5 | 80 |
| 6-9 | 6 |
| 10-12 | 4 |
| 13-17 | 10 |
| | 100 |
| | |
| *Reason for Grandchild's Placement* | |
| Parental alcohol and other drug abuse resulting in... | |
| Neglect | 36 |
| Abandonment | 24 |
| Physical abuse | 20 |
| Domestic violence | 14 |
| Fear | 6 |
| | 100 |
| *Contact with Parental Alcohol and Other Drug Abuser* | |
| Yes | 66 |
| No | 44 |
| | 100 |
| | |
| *Rurality* | |
| Farm town | 100 |

other drug abusing parent since they started taking care of the grand-child.

## Stressors

*Parenting Stress.* Scores for the overall parenting stress index was 84.25 (*SD = 22.76*) for married grandmothers and 72.64 (*SD = 15.61*) for the single-parent grandmothers. For the subscales, grandmothers' mean scores were 28.49 ($SD = 7.83$) for the dysfunctional parent-child interaction subscale, 31.44 ($SD = 10.61$), and 29.23 ($SD = 8.84$). The single-parent grandmothers' mean scores were 25.24 ($SD = 6.93$) for the difficult child subscale, 21.34 ($SD = 5.95$) for the dysfunctional parent-child interaction subscale, and 27.21 ($SD = 8.44$) for the parental distress subscale.

*Financial Stress.* The most talked about stressor was that of financial difficulties. Consistently, these grandparents expressed "esto es muy dificil para mi, porque yo no tengo mucho dinero. Yo no recibo seguro social ni otro dinero de gobierno." Another grandmother who was in contact with the substance abusing parent reported, "cuando mi hijo vino a visitar a mi nena, yo le di poco dinero; cual es mi responsibilidad?" Some grandparents confronted pressure of providing for parent in addition to the financial responsibility of the grandchild.

In some families, grandparents pointed out that their financial assistance for providing the much needed care to a grandchild was less than a foster parent would be paid for caring for the same child. Moreover, some felt it was not worth the time and energy of going into social and health care agencies to apply for help. Thus, in these type families social and health care for a growing child may become a critical issue because many grandparents raising grandchildren may not seek financial assistance. Instead, they attempt to manage the child's health needs out-of-pocket. This management strategy often forces grandparents to choose between a health maintenance visit for the grandchild, purchasing their own medication, or buying food for the family. The most necessary expense as viewed by these families was food and medical attention was secondary. However, the sacrifice of health care for food cost for the entire family places both grandchild and grandparents at further risk for illness.

Some of these elderly grandparents were still working when they assumed primary care for the grandchild. When asked, "have you had to make changes in your job or job responsibilities due to your child care responsibilities?" some grandmothers reported they quit their jobs to provide care for grandchildren who need care. This can be perceived as a negative experience because employment can contribute to one's independence and identity, provides dignity, income, and an opportunity for retirement.

*Inadequate Housing.* Grandchildren moving in with grandparents often caused crowding for these families in their present living space. Most of grandparents were living in what they considered to be small spaces and making room for a grandchild presented major obstacles, often leaving both child and grandparents with little privacy or personal space. This compounded both depressive reactions and anxiety reported by the grandmothers. This finding is consistent with previous studies (Jendrek, 1994; Musil, Youngblut, Ahn, & Curry, 2001) that have documented increased levels of stress when grandchildren co-reside with the grandparents. Nonetheless, some respondents in the present study reported that they liked having the grandchild move into their home. Some grandmothers said they "enjoyed the company" and the grandchild could help with instrumental activities of daily living, such as taking out the trash and cleaning the house. This finding was consistent with other research (Orel & Dupuy, 2003) that has looked at reciprocity and coping among grandparents who parent grandchildren. At the same time, feelings of being overwhelmed by the lack of quiet time and inadequate living space prevailed in these rural families.

*Social Isolation.* Social isolation and role restriction can lead to a sense of resentment associated with the loss of anticipated freedom from parental responsibilities. For example, while a grandparent may enjoy being a grandparent when the child visits for only a short time, when they take on the role of full-time parent, this infringes on their ability to perform the activities expected for this late stage of life. The following excerpt indicates that.

> *I like to cook and work in my garden and I used to do that with my neighbor, but now I'm too tired. I'm too old to be doing the childcare. I think my son forgot about me. I stay home all day and take care of her. I didn't think my son would not be around to raise her. I expected to be helping, but sometimes I just want to go out and enjoy the day. Now, I am too tired to go anywhere and I don't even go to Mass on Sunday anymore.*

There were reports of social isolation that were present due to a lack of transportation in the communities, but when grandparents assumed the care of their own child's children, social isolation grew twofold. Not only were the grandparents isolated, but the grandchildren were also isolated because the grandparents reported not having felt the need to deal with the hassles of trying to find transportation in rural areas. This is a tremendous problem across settings (Coward & Krout, 1998).

Grandmothers discussed their interaction with peers who did not have similar parenting responsibilities. Other older adults in the community were "much less likely to spend time with me now" that I am caring for my grandchild was echoed in the narratives of these grandparents. This contributed significantly to their social isolation. Another barrier to social connectedness was the role restrictions brought on by daily parenting tasks. Diaper washing, midnight feeding, infant and childhood illnesses can provoke hardship and aggravate an already stressful situation.

Grandparents shared their concerns about having to continue parenting for an indefinite period of time. Not knowing if the alcohol or other drug abusing parent was likely to discontinue use of substances or to return for the child with or without being off drugs, these grandparents lived in constant worry and despair. One grandmother commented, "I don't feel good going out for enjoyment, when I don't know if my own daughter is safe or if drugs have claimed her life. I wonder what will happen to my granddaughter if I am not here for her." Social isolation can also lead to psychosocial stress.

*Psychosocial Stress.* This group of grandmothers felt that language barriers create a disconnect for them in gaining access to the necessary information. They expressed concern about their need to become more knowledgeable about the impact that alcohol and other drug abuse can have on children as well as problems and solutions that currently exist but according to them, were less prevalent when they were parenting their own children (e.g., anxiety, depression, by products of acculturation). Furthermore, the women reported that they view their grandchildren as much more aggressive than they were accustomed to dealing with. They felt this might be related to the exposure to violence and other dysfunctional relationships promoted by substance abusing parents.

Additionally, grandparents who suddenly were confronted with health problems of grandchildren tended to minimize their own social and health care needs. A reoccurring theme for the participating grandmothers was "I would rather have the child healthy than me." The grandmothers felt it was a high priority to provide a better life for the grandchildren than the children's parents had provided. In many cases this meant grandmothers neglected their own health so that the children could be taken care of. One 72-year-old grandmother responded, "it's OK, I've had my time, ahora le voy a cuidar mis nietos."

In a very caring and concerned fashion, many of the grandparents believed that the grandchildren whom they were caring for suffered from bitterness and depression as a result of early childhood trauma, parental loss, and exposure to drugs and other substances. They acknowledged that a benefit to their parenting role is the opportunity to provide a loving and nurturing home for their grandchildren, as much as they possibly can. It was evident in this research that many of the Latino grandmothers had come to appreciate the role they were functioning in and as has been found in previous research (Cox, Brooks, & Valcarcel, 2000), were fulfilling traditional expectations and familial obligations.

## DISCUSSION

This study investigated stressors, sacrifices and service needs of grandparents as parent for grandchildren of parental alcohol and other drug abusers to describe the subjective perception of elderly Latino grandmothers in a rural community. Limitations to this study include the relatively small sample size and lack of a control group. The fact that the grandparents in this sample were poor, had low educational attainment, and were from farm communities raises questions about the generalizability of the results. However, the findings bring to bear particular issues of the applicability of data from samples that are not representative of communities like this rural elderly Latino population, which need to be addressed in order to extend alcohol and other drug abuse intervention.

The phenomenon of grandparents as parents can be one of grandparents often not knowing the whereabouts of the alcohol or other drug abusing parent but in other cases, grandparents provide assistance to the parent. Stress, sacrifices, and a great need for services are factors that complicate life for these families. Grandparents as parents sacrifice their time for relaxation and peer relationships; they sacrifice the limited financial resources, and they sacrifice their psychosocial well-being. Yet, findings from this study indicate that elderly Latino grandmothers manage to find positive and reciprocal aspects of the relationships with their grandchildren.

The identification of stressors as predictors of the ability to perform activities of daily living provides direction for intervention in rural communities. Single grandparent-headed families experienced more overall parenting stress than married grandmothers as parents in this study. Having a secondary care provider might ease the burden (Tennstedt, Crawford, & McKinlay, 1993) and make caregiving a bit less taxing on the elder, especially when alcohol and other drug abuse issues are present. Other studies have not looked specifically at marital status of grandparents in relation to substance abusing parents and its effects on grandchildren's care. However, previous research has compared grandmother caretakers to published norms and found grandparents' stress scores to be higher (Kelley, 1993). The more elevated level of stress was expected due to the challenges that grandparents face when parenting a grandchild. The increased psychosocial stress reported by the grandparents is of concern to practitioners given that increased stress is associated with the loss of ability to perform activities of daily living such as parenting tasks and physical health maintenance (Burnette, 1999c).

The context in which the care occurs should be explored for points of entry to support these families. When considering questions about the impact of parental alcohol and other drug abuse on grandparent-headed households, it is important to assess the specific characteristics for the living environment, whether the family has access to transportation, financial stability, less than adequate housing and respite for social interaction with peers. One 65-year-old grandmother remarked, "part of my stress would be gone if we could find a larger place to live in that was down that long dark road with no lights and no way to get to the store."

Particularly significant is the fact that family plays an important role in individuals' lives and provides a unique set of functions not met by formal organizations (Bullock, 2004). An evaluation of the contact that the grandparent has with the parental alcohol and other drug abuser may provide information on family functioning. For these rural grandmothers there was a range of stress-related references to the interaction with the child's parent. While some parents feared the presence of the alcohol or other drug abusing parent, others felt that the complete absence of the parent could negatively affect the child as well, impacting the psychosocial development of the child. Given the potential cost to family systems when they are compromised by alcohol and other drug abuse problems, there needs to be further examination of the risks and potential benefits associated with the presence versus absence of a substance abusing parent so that there are empirical data to inform directions and decisions about circumstances under which it might be prudent to encourage parental involvement and circumstance under which it might be better to invoke procedures designed to protect grandparents and grandchildren from potential harm associated with the presence of a substance abusing parent.

There is undoubtedly a need for creative interventions that support grandparents as parents who are affected by parental alcohol and other drug abuse. Individual stressor identified by these grandparents suggests that maneuvering through the educational, health care, and legal systems is a challenge. Consistent with other data (Cox, Brooks, & Valcarcel, 2000; Toledo et al., 2000) this research confirms that Latino grandparents may experience language barriers that interfere with their ability to access the support services they need. Also, elders may not have the energy to sit all day, waiting to be seen in agencies. For elders in the present study, this was further complicated when the dependent child had special health needs, which may have been exacerbated by their exposure to alcohol and other drug abuse. In some cases, the grandparent as parent was required to function as a case manager when the child was diagnosed with a chronic illness. When the grandparent was raising more than one grandchild with health or psychosocial problems, there was often competition for scarce family resources. Grandparents requested assistance with brokerage and advocacy within the health care and social welfare systems in order to meet their support needs and to provide safe and adequate care to the grandchildren they are raising. While these findings provide a description of stressor, sacrifices and service needs of grandmothers in a rural community, there continues to be a need for additional research on this topic.

## IMPLICATIONS FOR PRACTICE

Of the frameworks proposed for understanding the subjective perception of the impact that alcohol and other drug abuse has on the grandparents as parents in a rural Latino community, social adaptation was most useful in the present analyses. This approach recognizes the family diversity as a legitimate adaptation to the socioeconomic context. Increased contextual, familial, and individual dynamics among Latinos can be expected to influence the current and future way that we work with families. The time has come to add grandparents as parents to the agenda. Building upon research done with grandparents raising grandchildren and disenfranchised populations, the alcohol and other drug abuse research community needs to carefully consider a number of related issues so that there is an empirical database to inform public policy designed to minimize the impact of alcohol and other drug abuse on families.

It is noteworthy that grandparents were able and willing to express their concerns and share their perception of the impact of alcohol and other drug abuse on their families. This may be viewed as a dire need for assistance. Reaching out through research participation is one way of giving voice to their experiences. When considering the impact of paternal alcohol and other drug abuse on children, researchers need to move beyond concern about vertical transmission of alcohol and other drug abuse and document more clearly the ways in which chronic drug and alcohol use of substance abusing parents directly and indirectly affect development outcomes for children. Moving beyond the deficit model of the grandparent as parent phenomenon, practitioners must also acknowledge the strengths of extended families in taking up the charge of caring for their members as well as positive contributions that alcohol and other drug-abusing parents might make.

Health and social services agencies can reach out to rural elderly Latinos by involving community representatives in the intervention process and making culturally sound recommendation for practice and program development. Information should be made available in Spanish language, which will help to decrease barriers to service for this population. These efforts can assist in meeting the special needs of rural Latino grandparents raising grandchildren of alcohol and other drug abusing parents.

## REFERENCES

Adibin, R.R. (1995). *Parenting stress index. Professional manual* (3rd ed.). Odessa, FL: Psychological Assessment Resources.

Alderete, E., Vega, W.A., Kolody, B., & Aguilar-Gaxiola, S. (2000). Lifetime prevalence of and risk factors of psychiatric disorder among Mexican migrant farmworkers in California. *American Journal of Public Health, 90* (4), 608-614.

Amaro, H., & Russo, N.F. (1987). Hispanic women and mental health, *Psychology of Women Quarterly, 11*, 393-407.

Angel, R.J., Angel, J.L., Lee, G., & Markides, K.S. (1999). Age at migration and family dependency among older Mexican immigrants: Recent evidence from the Mexican American EPESE. *The Gerontologist, 39* (1), 59-65.

Anglin, M.D. (1990). Drug-abuse treatment to ameliorate negative family and childhood effects of parental drug use. In *Raising children for the twenty-first century* (pp. 325-331). Washington, DC: American Enterprise Institute.

Anhalt, H., & Klein, M. (1976). Drug abuse in junior high school populations. *American Journal of Drug and Alcohol Abuse, 3*, 589-603.

Applewhite, S.L. (1998). Culturally competent practice with elderly Latinos. In M. Delgado (Ed.), *Latino elders and the twenty-first century: Issues and challenges for culturally competent research and practice* (pp. 1-15). New York, NY: Haworth Press.

Becerra, R.M., & Shaw, D. (1988). *The Hispanic elderly: A research reference guide.* Lanham, MD: University Press of America.

Brown-Standridge, M.D., & Floyd, C.W. (2000). Healing bittersweet legacies: Revisiting contextual family therapy for grandparents raising grandchildren in crisis. *Journal of Marriage and Family Therapy, 26* (2), 185-197.

Bryson, K. (2001, November). *New Census Bureau data on grandparents raising grandchildren.* Paper presented at the 54th Annual Scientific meeting of the Geronotological Society of America, Chicago, IL.

Bullock, K. (2004). Family social support. In P.J. Bomar, 3rd ed. (Ed.), *Nurse and family health promotion: Concepts, research, assessment, and intervention*, pp. 142-161. St. Louis, MO: WB Saunders of Harcourt Health Sciences.

Bullock, K. (2001). Health family systems: The changing role of grandparents in rural America. *Education & Ageing, 16* (2), 163-178.

Burnette, D. (1999a). Social relationships of Latino grandparent caregivers: A role theory perspective. *The Gerontologist, 39* (1), 49-58.

Burnette, D. (1999b). Custodial grandparents in Latino families: Patterns of service use and predictors of unmet needs. *Social Work, 44* (1), 22-34.

Burnette, D. (1999c). Physical and emotional well-being of custodial grandparents in Latino families. *American Journal of Orthopsychiatry, 69* (3), 305-318.

Burton, L.M. (1992). Black grandparents rearing grandchildren of drug addicted parents: Stressors, outcomes, and social service needs. *The Gerontologist, 37,* 744-751.

Calderon, V., & Tennstedt, S. (1998). Ethnic differences in expression of caregiver burden. *Journal of Gerontological Social Work, 30* (1/2), 159-178.

Carlton-LaNey, I. (1992). Elderly Black farm women: A population at risk. *Social Work, 37* (6), 517-523.

Casper, L.M., & Bryson, K.R. (1998). *Co-resident grandparents and their grandchildren: Grandparent maintained families* (Population Division Working Paper No. 26). Washington, DC: U.S. Bureau of the Census. Retrieved July 31, 2001, from *http://www.census.gov/population/www/documentation/twps0026.html*

Chapa, J., & Valencia, R.R. (1993). Latino population growth, characteristics, demographic characteristics and educational stagnation: An examination of recent trends. *Hispanic Journal of Behavioral Science, 15,* 165-187.

Coward, R.T., & Krout, J.A. (1998). *Aging in rural settings: Life circumstances and distinctive features.* New York, NY: Springer.

Cox, C.B. (2002). Empowering African American custodial grandparents. *Social Work, 47* (1), 45-54.

Cox, C.B., Brooks, L.R., & Valcarcel, C. (2000). Culture and caregiving: A study of Latino grandparents. In C.B. Cox (Ed.), *To grandmother's house we go and stay: Perspectives on custodial grandparents* (pp. 218-232). New York, NY: Springer.

De La Rosa, M.R., Segal, B., & Lopez, R. (1999). *Conducting drug abuse research with minority populations: Advances and issues.* New York, NY: Haworth Press.

Delgado, M. (2002). Latinos and alcohol: Treatment considerations. *Alcoholism Treatment Quarterly, 20* (3/4), 187-192.

Delgado, M. (1998a). *Social services in Latino communities.* New York, NY: Haworth Press.

Delgado, M. (1998b). *Latino elders and the twenty-first century: Issues and challenges for culturally competent research and practice.* New York, NY: Haworth Press.

Fox, R.A., & Solis-Camara, P. (1997). Parenting of young children by fathers in Mexico and the United States. *Journal of Social Psychology, 137,* 489-495.

Fuller-Thomson, E., & Minkler, M. (2000). African American grandparents raising grandchildren: A national profile of demographic and health characteristics. *Health & Social Work, 25* (2), 109-118.

Gibson, P.A. (2002). African American grandmothers as caregivers: Answering the call to help their grandchildren. *Families in Society: The Journal of Contemporary Human Services, 83* (1), 35-43.

Gilbert, M.J. (1987). Alcohol consumption patterns in immigrant and later generation Mexican women. *Hispanic Journal of Behavioral Sciences, 9* (3), 299-313.

Gorman-Smith, D., Tolan, P.H., Henry, D.B., & Leventhal, A. (2001). Predictors of participation in a family-focused prevention intervention for substance abuse. *Psychology of Addictive Behaviors, 16* (4), S55-S64.

Gruber, K.J., Fleetwood, T.W., & Herring, M.W. (2001). In-home continuing care services for substance-affected families: The Bridge Program. *Social Work, 46* (3), 267-277.

Hayslip, B., Jr., & Goldberg-Glen, R. (2000). *Grandparents raising grandchildren: Theoretical, empirical, and clinical perspectives.* New York, NY: Springer.

Hirshorn, B.A., Van Meter, M.J., & Brown, D.R. (2000). When grandparents raise grandchildren due to substance abuse: Responding to a uniquely destabilizing factor. In B. Hayslip, Jr. & R. Goldberg-Glen (Eds.), *Grandparents raising grandchildren: Theoretical, empirical, and clinical perspectives* (pp. 269-287). New York: Springer.

Jendrek, M.P. (1994). Granparents who parent their grandchildren: Circumstances and decisions. *The Geronotologist, 34,* 206-216.

Jessor, R. (1976). Predicting time of onset of marijuana use: A developmental study of high school youth. *Journal of Consulting Clinical Psychology, 44,* 125-134.

Kandel, D.B., & Logan, J.A. (1984). Patterns of drug use from adolescents to young adulthood: Periods of risks for initiation, continued use, and discontinuation. *American Journal of Public Health, 74,* 660-666.

Kearney, M.H., Murphy, S., & Rosenbaum, M. (1994). Mothering on crack: A grounded theory analysis. *Social Science and Medicine, 38,* 351-361.

Kelley, S.J. (1993). Caregiver stress in grandparents raising grandchildren. *IMAGE: Journal of Nursing Scholarship, 25,* 331-337.

Marsigalia, F.F., & Daley, J.M. (2002). Latinos participating in multiethnic coalitions to prevent substance abuse: A case study. *Journal of Human Behavior in the Social Environment, 5* (3/4), 97-121.

McMahon, T.J., Winkel, J.D., Suchman, N.E., & Luthar, S.S. (2002). Drug dependence, parenting responsibilities, and treatment history: Why doesn't mom go for help? *Drug and Alcohol Dependence, 65,* 105-114.

Minkler, M., & Roe, K.M. (1993). *Grandmothers as caregivers: Raising children of the crack epidemic.* Newbury Park, CA: Sage.

Minkler, M., Fuller-Thomson, E., Miller, D., & Driver, D. (1997). Depression in grandparents raising grandchildren. *Archives of Family Medicine, 6,* 445-452.

Musil, C.M., Youngblut, J.M., Ahn, S., & Curry, V.L. (2001). Parenting stress: A comparison of grandmother caretakers and mothers. *Journal of Mental Health and Aging, 8* (3), 197-210.

Napier, T.L., Bachtel, D.C., & Carter, M.V. (1983). Factors associated with illegal drug use in rural Georgia. *Journal of Drug Education, 13,* 119-140.

National Institute on Drug Abuse (1990). *National household survey on drug abuse: Highlights 1988.* Department of Health and Human Services (DHHS) Publication No. ADM 90-1681. Washington, DC: Government Printing Office.

NC Office of Minority Health (1999). *Latina reproductive health in North Carolina: Demographics, health status, and programs.* Division of Public Health. NC Department of Health & Human Services. Raleigh, NC.

Orel, N.A., & Dupuy, P. (2003) Grandchildren as auxiliary caregivers for grandparents with cognitive and/or physical limitations: Coping strategies and ramifications. *Child Study Journal, 32* (4), 193-213.

Parke, R.D. (2002). Substance-abusing fathers: Descriptive process & methodological perspectives. *Addiction, 97* (9), 1118-1119.

Philleo, J., & Brisbane, F.L. (1995). *Cultural competence for social worker: A guide for alcohol and other drug abuse prevention professionals working with ethnic/racial communities* (pp. 43-67). CSPA Cultural Competence Series 4. U.S. Department of Health and Human Services. Pub No. (SMA)95-3075, Rockville, MD.

Poindexter, C.C., & Linsk, N.L. (1999). "I'm just glad that I'm here": Stories of seven African-American grandmothers. *Journal of Gerontological Social Work, 32* (1), 63-81.

Pruchno, R.A., & McKenney, D. (2002). Psychological well-being of black and white grandmothers raising grandchildren: Examination of a two-factor model. *Journal of Geronotology: Psychological Science, 57B (5),* 444-452.

Purnell, L.D. (1998). Mexican Americans. In L.D. Purnell & B.J. Paulanka (Eds.), *Transcultural health care: A culturally competent approach* (pp. 397-421). Philadelphia: F.A. Davis Company.

Roe, K.M., Minkler, M., & Barnwell, R.S. (1994). The assumption of caregiving: Grandmothers raising the children of the crack cocaine epidemic. *Qualitative Health Research, 4,* 281-303.

Roe, K.M., Minkler, M., Saunders, F., & Thomson, G.E. (1996). Health of grandmothers raising children of the crack cocaine epidemic. *Medical Care, 34,* 1072-1084.

Soriano, F.I. (1993). AIDS and intravenous drug use among Hispanics in the U.S.: Considerations for prevention efforts. In R.S. Mayers & B.L. Kail (Eds.), *Hispanic substance abuse* (pp. 131-144).

Sotomayor, M. (1989). The Hispanic elderly and the intergenerational family. *Journal of Children in Contemporary Society, 20* (3/4), 55-65.

Stoller, E.P. (1998). Families of elderly rural Americans. In R.T. Coward & J.A. Krout (Eds.), *Aging in rural settings: Life circumstances and distinctive features* (pp. 127-146). New York, NY: Springer.

Suchman, N.E., & Luthar, S.S. (2000). Maternal addiction, child maladjustment, and sociodemographic context: Implications for parenting behaviors. *Addiction, 95,* 1417-1428.

Tennstedt, S.L., Crawford, S.L., & McKinlay, J.B. (1993). Is family care on the decline? A longitudinal investigation of the substitution of formal long-term care services for informal care. *The Milbank Quarterly, 71,* 601-624.

Toledo, J.R., Hayslip, Jr., B., Emick, M.A., Toledo, C., & Henderson, C.E. (2000). Cross-cultural differences in custodial grandparenting. In B. Hayslip, Jr. & R.

Goldberg-Glen (Eds.), *Grandparents raising grandchildren: Theoretical, empirical, and clinical perspectives* (pp. 107-123). New York: NY, Springer.

U.S. Bureau of the Census (2002). Population Trends. Retrieved September 20, 2002, from *http://www.census.gov/population/*

Vega, W.A. (1990). Hispanic families in the 1980s: A decade of research. *Journal of Marriage and the Family, 52,* 1015-1024.

Whitley, D.M., Kelley, S.J., & Sipe, T.A. (2001). Grandmothers raising grandchildren: Are they at increased risk of health problem? *Health & Social Work, 26* (2), 105-114.

Zambrana, R.E., & Aguirre-Molina, M. (1987). Alcohol abuse prevention among Latino adolescents: A strategy for intervention. *Journal of Youth & Adolescence, 16* (2), 97-113.

Chapter 8

# Creating Circulos del Cuidado for AOD Latino Juvenile Offenders

Edward Pabon, PhD

**SUMMARY.** Latin youth and their families are increasingly disproportionately represented in the juvenile justice system. Such disparities will continue until Latino communities develop natural alternatives such as Circulos del Cuidado (Circles of Care) within their communities to prevent and/or reduce involvement with the juvenile justice system. *[Article copies available for a fee from The Haworth Document Delivery Service: 1-800-HAWORTH. E-mail address: <docdelivery@haworthpress.com> Website: <http://www.HaworthPress.com> © 2005 by The Haworth Press, Inc. All rights reserved.]*

**KEYWORDS.** Latino youth, juvenile justice, intervention

Latino youth and their families are increasingly disproportionately represented in the juvenile justice system. Harsh and disparate treatment at all stages of the justice system (including arrest, detention,

Edward Pabon is Assistant Professor of Social Work, Marywood University, College of Health & Human Services, School of Social Work, 2640 Station Avenue, Campbell Hall Building, Center Valley, PA 18034.

[Haworth co-indexing entry note]: "Creating Circulos del Cuidado for AOD Latino Juvenile Offenders." Pabon, Edward. Co-published simultaneously in *Alcoholism Treatment Quarterly* (The Haworth Press, Inc.) Vol. 23, No. 2/3, 2005, pp. 131-147; and: *Latinos and Alcohol Use/Abuse Revisited: Advances and Challenges for Prevention and Treatment Programs* (ed: Melvin Delgado) The Haworth Press, Inc., 2005, pp. 131-147. Single or multiple copies of this article are available for a fee from The Haworth Document Delivery Service [1-800-HAWORTH, 9:00 a.m. - 5:00 p.m. (EST). E-mail address: docdelivery@haworthpress.com].

doi:10.1300/J020v23n02_08

waiver to adult criminal court, and sentencing) is usually a grim reality for many Latinos. Racial and ethnic disparities in the system, compounded by an unprecedented rate of construction of new juvenile facilities, jails and prisons across the country, continues to spell trouble for Latino youth, who are part of the largest and fastest-growing racial/ethnic group in the United States.

Such disparities will continue until Latino communities develop natural alternatives such as Circulos del Cuidado (Circles of Care) within their communities to prevent and/or reduce involvement with the juvenile justice system. Using the preference of Latinos for informal supports in help seeking, the Circulos del Cuidado is a meeting of all family members, child welfare/juvenile justice officials, members of the community, such as resource and support persons, and other persons involved with the family to plan for the care and protection of the youth and the family involved with the juvenile justice system.

## *CULTURAL INSENSITIVITY OF THE JUSTICE SYSTEM*

Unfortunately, the absence of comprehensive data makes it impossible to determine the full extent of disparate and punitive treatment of Latino youth at key decision points in the justice system, or to fully develop more comprehensive and effective policies to remedy the disparities. Data available are limited because states do not routinely and systematically collect data that separate Latino youth from White youth, or distinguish among Latino youth of Mexican, Caribbean, Central American, or South American ancestry. The failure to collect separate data on Latino youth also inflates the incarceration rate of non-Hispanic White youth, further masking disparities in confinement of all youth of color.

Disparate treatment of Latino youth manifests itself in numerous ways. In some states, Latino children and youth in the child welfare system are overrepresented in out-of-home placements, with percentages in placement as high as 56% in New Mexico, 32% in Connecticut, 31% in California and Texas, and 27% in Arizona (Villarruel & Walker, 2002).

Latino youth also are transferred from juvenile court to adult criminal court at greater rates than White youth. Anti-gang statutes in many states impose dramatically higher penalties on youth who courts presume to be "gang members." The justice system often relies on assumptions about which youth are involved in gangs, based on racial and ethnic stereotypes about Latino youth. As a result, Latino youth who have no involvement whatsoever with gangs can nevertheless face prosecution and long mandatory minimum sentences if convicted.

Immigrant youth, the majority of whom are Latino, face severe hardships if they come to the attention of the Immigration and Naturalization Service (INS). Oftentimes they experience psychological trauma and long periods of detention in jails and other facilities, as well as possible deportation and permanent separation from their families. Further, once Latino youth are taken into custody, their parents may be afraid to have contact with authorities if the parents are not U.S. citizens and may be subject to deportation. Even those Latino parents who are U.S. citizens may resist invasions of their privacy and having to prove their citizenship. In addition, it may be difficult or, in some cases, impossible for youth in migrant families, such as farm worker families, to comply with probation requirements, turning minor misbehaviors into serious violations.

In addition, most youth who enter drug abuse treatment do so through the juvenile justice system once they have had a run-in with the law. The consequences of the juvenile alcohol-crime cycle are severe. AOD use among juvenile delinquents appears to be strongly related to other social and psychological problems, including lowered school performance, poor family relationships, and increased interactions with AOD using peers (Howell, Krisberg, Hawkins, & Wilson, 1995). AOD use also appears to be associated with a number of delinquent behaviors. A high proportion of juveniles (likely the majority) processed by the juvenile court have recently used illegal substances, and juvenile AOD use appears to be related to recurring, chronic, and violent delinquency that continues into adulthood (Demo, Shemwell, Guida, Schmeider, Pacheco, & Seeberger, 1998). The juvenile justice system is, therefore, a viable point of entry for a service program designed to break the juvenile alcohol-crime cycle, especially among minority youth.

Very few juvenile justice jurisdictions provide appropriate substance abuse treatment services for youth. Thornberry et al. found that treatment for adolescent substance offenders was available in less than 40 percent of the 3,000 public and private juvenile detention, correctional, and shelter facilities across the United States (Thornberry, Tolnay, Flanagan, & Glynn, 1991). Jurisdictions that provide treatment generally limit access to support group services, such as Alcoholics Anonymous (AA) and Narcotics Anonymous (NA), as well as AOD testing (Schonberg, 1993). While a few settings conduct individual or group sessions for substance-abusing juveniles, these facilities do not generally conduct comprehensive treatment needs assessments or plan and carry out individualized treatment programs along a continuum of care. New interventions within the system are needed to address these deficiencies; such programming must be clearly aware of and logically incorporate the etiology, correlates, and consequences of the alcohol-crime cycle.

As more adolescents of diverse racial and ethnic backgrounds are identified to be in need of drug abuse treatment services, questions arise about the degree to which treatments need to be tailored for specific genders, or ethnic or cultural groups. Limited research has examined the effectiveness of culturally congruent assessment and treatment services on engagement, and for only a few cultural groups. Comparatively little research attention is given to gender, cultural, ethnic, and linguistic sensitivity and specificity in treatment and other health services. The extant research that does address these issues suggests that there are cultural differences in the patterns of comorbidity observed among drug abusing adolescents and in their treatment service needs (Robbins, Kumar, Walker-Barnes, Feaster, Briones, & Szapocznik, 2002).

The understanding that adolescents who abuse drugs have problems and treatment needs unique from those of other populations raises the question of just who the providers delivering those treatment services should be. Given the many different systems that influence the lives of drug abusing youth (e.g., family, education, mental health, medical, welfare, criminal justice), treatment practitioners need both knowledge of these systems and skill in navigating them. Few studies have examined the adolescent treatment workforce (Pond, Aguiree-Molina, & Orleans, 2002), but there is evidence of a growing disparity between the demographic profiles of treatment providers and the adolescents they treat (Northwest Frontier Addiction Technology Transfer Center, 2000). These findings raise questions about the extent to which the cadre of practitioners currently treating adolescent drug abusers is sufficiently prepared to do so.

Amidst the discussion of treatment modalities and effectiveness, it is important to recognize that while knowledge of general effectiveness exists to some degree, there is very little information on the relationship between treatment program outcomes among different ethnic/cultural groups. Interventions at any point of system contact (diversion, disposition, and sentencing) may have differential effects on adolescents based on their ethnic association. Ethnicity can affect family relationships, achievement orientations, and perceptions of authority structures and treatment providers. Care must be taken to address considerations of ethnicity in developing interventions that are effective with adolescents from a broad range of backgrounds or that meet the specific needs of a given population.

When we overly rely on professional helpers, formal agencies, and system solutions, we may fail to create strategies fully relevant to specific communities or we may fail to produce experiences that result in increased self-efficacy and empowerment among families seeking help. In addition, a lack of partnership between formal services and informal support systems may constrain the opportunities for families to receive support on a 24-hour, seven-days-a-week basis. Families may be left to seek out support from relatives and neighbors who may not have the skills and resources necessary to respond to a crisis. Professionals may experience frustration at setbacks that families experience after office hours, when professionals are unable to respond. Often, there is a significant disconnect between formal and informal systems, between formal service providers and natural helpers.

## USING THE "COMMUNITY"

A culturally competent system of children and youth care must acknowledge and incorporate, at all levels, respect for the unique, culturally defined needs of various client populations; the importance of culture as a predominant force in shaping behaviors and values; the view of natural systems (e.g., family, community, church) as primary mechanisms of support for clients; the recognition of the importance of sociocultural, linguistic, and national heterogeneity in the care and treatment of clients; the acknowledgement that people are served in varying degrees by their natural systems; and the recognition that concepts such as "family" and "community" are different for various cultures and even for subgroups within cultures.

Many community service initiatives have defined community primarily in terms of geography, ignoring the very vibrant sense of community that exists in personal networks of relationships. In doing so they may, in reality, be indistinguishable from existing service practices, failing to establish meaningful roles for community members in service interventions. It is the deeply interpersonal nature of such interrelations that give the collective community its character and strength. The greater the abstraction in defining community, the further it is removed from interdependency and the locus of existing informal social control. That is why it is important for community service to encourage and create community, as a perception of connectedness to an individual or group, in its efforts to respond to and prevent social problems.

"Circles" are currently emerging as a process and structure to enhance local community involvement in matters of justice. Circles amount to a partnership arrangement between governmental officials, the family, and members of the community in acknowledging that decisions affecting families are better arrived at by respecting the integrity of the family unit, focusing on strengthening family and community supports, and creating opportunities for parents and other adults, including extended family members, to feel responsible for their children.

The use of circles for structuring communication and decision-making is likely as ancient as humankind (Baldwin, 1994). In Native American cultures the use of talking circles is part of an oral tradition handed down through the generations. Talking circles may serve a number of purposes, not the least being simply gathering the people.

For the participant among these cultures, the circle emerges out of shared living and embodies both power and mystery. While viewed as an old way of involving community members in dispute resolution, circles have been recently revitalized, if not repackaged, as another option within the developing restorative justice paradigm. Use of circles has generated considerable interest and a fair number of passionate adherents. Proponents speak of the "sacred quality," of the "power," of the "inclusiveness," of the "restorative nature" of the circle.

Though testimonies prevail, little descriptive information is available about how circles function to meet the purpose of restoring justice and how the circle experience is received by a variety of participants. The tradition of using circles to assist in resolving disputes and conflict is lodged deeply within native cultures in Canada and the United States. Since the 1980s in the Yukon, First Nation people and local justice officials have developed partnerships between communities and formal justice agencies to build shared responsibility for handling crime problems through Community Peacemaking Circles (Stuart, 1996, 1997). Communities in Manitoba have introduced circles of several types into their response to sex offenders, their victims, families, and community (Lajeunesse & Associates Ltd., 1996). Community leaders of the Mille Lacs Indian Reservation in Minnesota have worked with criminal justice officials to employ circle sentencing for selected cases in their community (Adams, 1998). Many other jurisdictions are also using some form of circle involvement or exploring its use to enhance community/neighborhood involvement and stake in criminal justice, to provide victims with a safe setting in which to be heard, and to offer opportunities for offenders to own their actions and participate in constructing meaningful ways of being held accountable (Bazemore & Griffiths, 1997; Bazemore & Umbreit, 1999).

Circles can take many forms and can occur at most any place in the justice process. Circles of understanding, healing circles (for offender and family, for victim and family, for offender, victim and community), sentencing circles and review of sentence compliance circles are just some mentioned in the literature. Each of these will have different purposes and the structure and process may vary some. Circles, as described in the literature, incorporate many of the components of reform efforts of the past decades: a strong emphasis upon local community member participation, making the circle community based; bringing victim and offender together in face to face interaction as does victim/offender mediation; and involving victim and offender family members and friends such as in family/group conferencing. And yet proponents of circles purport to do more by reaching back to native traditions of doing justice which predate Western criminal justice, by explicitly empowering each individual in the circle as an equal, and by explicitly lifting up the relationship between justice and the physical, emotional, and spiritual dimensions of individuals in the context of community and culture (Stuart, 1996, 1997; Lajeunesse & Associates, Ltd., 1996).

Very little descriptive or evaluative research has been done on the use of circles within the justice process. Training materials are available which provide descriptions of how circles are to function in theory (Stuart, 1997). The most substantial research on circles in the justice process was conducted in Manitoba where "healing circles" were used to work with sex abuse victims and their victimizers, their respective families and the community at large (Lajeunesse & Associates, Ltd., 1996). Circles were held with victimizers and their families, with victims and their families, and for sentencing (these circles included community members as well as the families and representatives of the formal justice system), and review of sentence compliance. Numerous other treatment/support healing circles were also available for specific groups, e.g., victims, victimizers, men, women, children. These circles were established in the Hollow Water First Nation community. Its relative isolation and homogeneity both enhanced and impaired the work of circles.

Results from this effort to develop a partnership whereby communities would take on a much larger role in the justice process than typical were mixed. Some participants reported benefiting immensely from the circle process. Having a voice and stake in justice outcomes, being understood, experiencing strengthened commitment to change and healing, mutual respect, and renewed community/cultural pride were cited as benefits of participation. Lack of privacy, difficulty of working with family and close friends, embarrassment, unprofessionalism, and religious conflict were cited by others as negative aspects of the circle process (Lajaeunesse & Associates, Ltd., 1996).

Little additional research seems to be available. Stuart makes reference to an unpublished recidivism study in the Kwanlin Dun Community which reported an eighty percent drop in repeat serious offenses (Stuart, 1997). In that same piece, Stuart makes a strong point that circle programs ought to be evaluated on their broader objectives as well as on the more traditional criminal justice measures such as recidivism. Many of those broader objectives have to do with community building and empowerment of community members (Stuart, 1996, 1997).

## *CREATING CIRCLES OF CARE*

For the Latino population, providing services means the utilization of a preference toward people and persons in their interpersonal relationships over concepts and ideas as vehicles to promote therapeutic engagement and relationship-building. Rogler, Malgady, Costantino and Blumenthal (1987) suggest that culturally sensitive services for Latinos must be reviewed with three considerations in mind: the accessibility of traditional treatments; the selection and altering of a traditional treatment according to perceived features of Latino culture; and the extraction of elements from Latino culture for use as an innovative treatment tool. Practice techniques, which enhance treatment services for the Latino individual and family, may be classified into three broad groupings: family, community-group, and individual. As such, effective engagement with Latino youngsters and families must incorporate an understanding of cultural influences on behavior patterns, especially toward the client-service provider relationship, targets of intervention, resource preference, and geographic location of services.

Clements (1988) has observed that treatment strategies must build the necessary community structures and involve as many informal supports as possible. In line with this assertion, services directed to the Latino community require attention not only to the importance of the family, but also involve the inclusion of other extended family members and institutions. As seen above, Latino help-seeking behavior patterns follow a course from family to government and public social service agencies as a last resort.

The Latino family is an extended one, built on strong ties to family members outside the nuclear family, as well as to persons outside the biological family through "fictive kinship." For the service provider, the extended or "fictive kinship" can provide a natural support system for the client in reinforcing the service provider's work.

And after the family, the church and the neighborhood can provide the service provider with a source of emotional and economic support for the client. The church can play an important role in providing the service provider with another natural support system for the client, but it can also assist in screening and channeling outside programs attempting to gain access to the local community and its population, including the service provider's client.

The barrio and its institutions (e.g., neighborhood grocery store, beauty parlors, restaurants, etc.) provides a means for information to be spread rapidly, where favors can be exchanged, and where social pressure can be brought to bear upon residents. In addition, according to Levitt (1995), owners of Latino establishments are motivated by a sense of social responsibility, as well as economic motives. This sense translates into providing culturally appropriate help for those customers in need, including financial assistance, counseling or advice, and information on formal and informal resources for help. Delgado (1996), in a study of Puerto Rican grocery stores and restaurants, identified eight key roles these institutions can play in the life of the community that extends beyond the selling of food: (1) providing credit; (2) cashing checks; (3) providing community-related news and information; (4) providing information from the homeland; (5) counseling customers in distress; (6) providing information about and referral to social service agencies; (7) assisting in filling out or interpreting government forms; and (8) providing cultural connectedness to the homeland through the selling of videos, publications, and so forth. Consequently, Latino businesses take on the role of nontraditional social service centers.

# Pathways of Help-Seeking

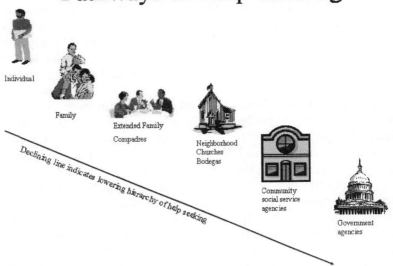

Individual

Family

Extended Family
Compadres

Neighborhood
Churches
Bodegas

*Declining line indicates lowering hierarchy of help seeking*

Community
social service
agencies

Government
agencies

Nontraditional settings are an indigenous source of support and are a place where individuals can gather to purchase a product or service or congregate for social purposes. These settings can facilitate conversation and the exchange of concerns and advice, minimizing the stigma for those seeking assistance. Exchange of advice and assistance is mutual; these settings are generally staffed by individuals who share the same ethnic, socioeconomic, and other key factors (i.e., religion, gender) maximizing psychological, geographical and cultural access and have a primary role that incorporates being a "helper." Their accessibility to the community makes these institutions excellent settings for collaboration with juvenile justice organizations. They can help distribute public education information, make referrals, perform crisis intervention, provide close supervision, help to interpret correspondence for non-English speaking clients, and fulfill other important roles.

The principle of engaging, linking and supporting formal services and informal supports to work in partnership in a community-based system of care begins with the acknowledgment that families and neighbors historically have provided critical supports to one another in a myriad of informal ways. When family members first recognize that they cannot solve a health or mental health problem by themselves, they typically turn first to family, friends, neighbors, or co-workers. The instinct to seek help from people close to us or provide help to those in our own family or community has been evident in areas such as birthing children, rearing and protecting children, providing shelter and meals, celebrating achievements and holidays, and sharing grieving over the loss of loved ones. Informal supports also play a critical role in supporting personal development and in coping with a significant change in family life, such as separation or divorce. This capacity for mutual support and the practice of providing informal supports by natural helpers in neighborhoods are essential to child and family well-being.

The concept of creating "Circulos del Cuidado" is a front-line practice change strategy with the objective to form professional/natural helper partnerships. It aims to increase the capacity to reach families that have been underrepresented in our formal systems of support and involve them in meaningful ways. It is a family-centered culturally competent, individualized process which supports the planning and co-ordinating of services and all helping efforts. Through the process, participants are acknowledged as leaders in their community, learning together with professional service providers diverse ways of sustaining a neighborhood system of care.

The circle process is value driven. The centrality of values is under-scored in the opening and closing of circles and often in the selection of a centerpiece or talking piece. Frequently mentioned values include: respect, humility, compassion, trust, hope, honesty, truth, gentleness, acceptance, flexibility, community, forgiveness, love, caring, integrity, openness, listening, sharing. This list is by no means exhaustive.

Participation in a circle is voluntary. Those engaged in conflict, those referred to the circle by the police or other authorities must choose to participate freely. Because the circle is not a fact finding body, any referred offender must admit guilt or acknowledge causing harm as part of applying to a circle.

Each individual has an equal opportunity to participate and is equally responsible for process and outcome. Repeatedly, circle conveners assure participants that there are "no experts" in the circle. Each person, by virtue of honoring the talking piece, has a right to speak and to be listened to. Participants should enter the circle with an open heart and an open mind. A corollary to this is not focusing on outcome. Appropriate outcomes will emerge from a process when individuals openly hear one another in a non-judgmental manner. A common refrain was that we must "think from the heart in order to discover how to resolve conflict."

Personal story is at the core of connectedness and conflict resolution. Individuals are encouraged to share their stories of joy and pain. Victims have the opportunity to speak to the emotional impact of crime and loss. Offenders have the opportunity to talk about what led to their own behavior and of their remorse. Community folks may speak to how crime impacts their own sense of safety and belonging. Many circle keepers and community representatives indicated that it is a "sacred opportunity to be present to really listen to another person's story."

The circle is a sacred space containing power greater than the sum of the individuals. Circles deal holistically with people and their problems. Behavioral, cognitive, emotional and spiritual dimensions are addressed. It is expected that participation in circles will lead to personal transformation and empathic responses to others which underpins universal spirituality (Pranis, 2000). Opening and closing rituals heighten this value-driven dimension.

The circle process is inclusive of all interests. It is crucial for a circle to hear from offender and victim, neighbors and justice system representatives. Any decisions made by the circle are made by consensus. What is said in the circle stays in the circle. Circle keepers remind circle participants of the need for confidentiality at the opening of nearly every circle. People are asked to speak their truth. Many find that they say more in the circle that they had originally planned on saying.

The "treatment theory" underlying the program depicts the process of human development as a reciprocal interchange between the individual and "nested concentric structures" that mutually influence one another (Freire, 1996). Extrafamilial systems, such as school, work, peer and even community and cultural institutions, are seen as interconnected with the individual and his or her family. The choice of treatment modality rests on adaptation and integration from pragmatic, problem-focused treatments that have at least some empirical support with Latino populations (Szapocznik & Fein, 1995).

The concept rests with the initial consensus regarding the identification of key natural supporters within the family or neighborhood network and the nature of the problems. Neighborhood facilitators would be encouraged to develop treatment strategies that are present focused and action oriented, targeting specific and well-defined problems. Support systems would be assessed early in the treatment process and extensive effort goes toward the development of networks, if these are insufficient.

The neighborhood natural facilitators would be responsible for surrounding at-risk families and youngsters who come to the attention of juvenile justice officials with a circle of care consisting of families and extra-family members, neighborhoods, and formal neighborhood representatives to assist the family (Umbreit, 2001). These neighborhood empowerment circles, which would be unique to each family, assumes that people gain control over their lives by increasing their participation in their community and society, by identifying and analyzing the social and historical roots to their problems, envisioning alternatives and acting to overcome the obstacles to social change, and by making social and personal changes. Most meetings would occur in the home, school, neighborhood, or community and would be accessible 24 hours a day and 7 days a week via cellular communication.

The key elements of the neighborhood empowerment circles concept are that:

- Social institutions can play important roles, but the process is centered on the community context of the situation.
- A wide net can be thrown to engage points of support of assistance and gather all relevant knowledge.
- Potential contributions can be expected even from those who are part of the problem, including at-risk family members and peers. There is an assumption that everyone has something to offer.
- Multiple issues can be dealt with at once. The approach recognizes that the issues interact with one another and cannot be effectively dealt with in isolation.
- Addressing issues is a shared responsibility. Taking individual responsibility in a community context, i.e., individuals identify specific acts they can take which fit with others' actions for a longer common good.
- Addressing personal, family, neighbor, and community issues require democratic participation in community decisions and in enhancing community health.
- Individuals recognize that there is mutual responsibility in that their well-being depends upon the well-being of all.
- The process provides an avenue for concrete individual action which increases understanding of broader social policy issues.
- The outcome is not just the creation of a solution to an individual problem but increased community capacity to support its members.
- The process also humanizes what are otherwise abstract issues of social policy.

The circles of care would be guided by a framework which emphasizes (1) group members shaping their own curriculum to address the problems they identify; (2) group members defining problems and solutions as they experience them, not only as experts define them; (3) group members have strengths, abilities, and knowledge to share and learn from each other; and (4) participants are co-learners creating a new understanding together. The value of the neighborhood empowerment circle format for discussion, brainstorming or problem solving includes:

- Share leadership, equality–Placing everyone in a circle minimizes structural distinctions between "teacher" and "learner" and sets a tone of equal participation and equal capacity to teach and learn among all participants.
- Visual contact among all participants at all times–In a circle no one is looking at anyone else's back. It is easier to listen and hear when there are direct sight and sound lines among participants.
- Focus–The structure of the circle focuses attention on the participants and task of the circle and reduces distractions.
- Connection–The circle links all participants with one another encouraging a sense of shared effort or common purpose.
- Respect/accountability–Because everyone in a circle can see one another encouraging a sense of shared effort or common purpose.
- Input and participation from all–Use of the technique of going around the circle providing each person with a chance to speak ensures that everyone has an opportunity to be heard and reduces domination of discussion by a small number of people.
- Inclusion–In a circle no one feels isolated or left out.

The natural network of supports in a Latino community would be used for early identification and treatment engagement. Outreach to neighborhood shops, businesses such as bodegas, and informal helpers yield many referrals for services. Moreover, identifying and contacting key informers in a community yield informal leaders who broker the natural supports in a neighborhood. Nontraditional settings are an indigenous source of support and are a place where individuals can gather to purchase a product or service or congregate for social purposes. These settings can facilitate conversation and the exchange of concerns and advice, minimizing the stigma for those seeking assistance. Exchange of advice and assistance is mutual; these settings are generally staffed by individuals who share the same ethnic, socioeconomic, and other key factors (i.e., religion, gender) maximizing psychological, geographical and cultural access and have a primary role that incorporates being a "helper." Their accessibility to the community makes these institutions excellent settings for collaboration. They can help distribute public education information, make referrals, perform crisis intervention, provide close supervision, help to interpret correspondence for non-English speaking clients, and fulfill other important roles (Delgado & Santiago, 1998).

The ultimate goal of the prevention and intervention strategies is the promotion of treatment generalization and long-term maintenance of therapeutic change. As such, each program component must involve collaboration, with both strong participant involvement and coordination of support services. Thus, treatment strategies would emphasize the development of skills that are to be used in the natural environment, and encourage work with key supporters and family members to increase their capacity to develop and implement appropriate solutions to problems that enhance the family's link with neighbor and community resources.

## *CREATING ALTERNATIVES*

The increasingly disproportionate representation of Latino youth in the juvenile justice system continues to spell trouble for these youth, who are part of the largest and fastest-growing racial/ethnic group in the United States. Most youth who enter the juvenile justice system appear to also have a need for alcohol and other drug abuse treatment. The consequences of the juvenile alcohol-crime cycle are severe. The juvenile justice system is, therefore, a viable point of entry for a service program designed to break the juvenile alcohol-crime cycle, especially among minority youth.

Given the expanding role of ethnic minorities in society and the problems that minority groups experience in relation to traditional juvenile justice services, alternative approaches capable of addressing the needs of cultural minorities need to be developed, validated, and disseminated across systems of juvenile justice. However, these approaches will continue to be unresponsive to the needs of minority clients, especially Latino youngsters, if they do not address the issue that juvenile justice service providers and Latino clients have different expectations and agendas as to treatment assessment, engagement, and practice. Any system of care should be capable of delivering culturally relevant services to its client population. There is a pressing need to take new directions that are culturally appropriate when providing services to Latino clients.

The core idea of the Circulos del Cuidado (Circles of Care) service approach is a meeting of all family members, juvenile justice officials, other persons involved with the family and the youngster, and interested community neighbors to plan for the care and protection of Latino youngsters at risk for deeper penetration into the juvenile justice system in terms of prevention and intervention. Circles amounts to a partnership arrangement between the state, represented by juvenile justice officials, the family, members of the family, and members of the community, such as resource and support persons, with each party expected to play an important role in planning and providing services to prevent and/or curtail deeper penetration of the youngster into the juvenile justice system. While building on the perspective that services directed to the Latino community require attention not only to the importance of the family, the concept also involves the inclusion of other extended family members and institutions. Thus, it involves the use of the natural supports seen as preference in Latino help-seeking behavior patterns.

## REFERENCES

Adams, J. (1999). *Circles of justice*, Star Tribune, August 18.

Baldwin, C. (1994). *Calling the Circle*. Newberg, Or.: Swan Raven & Company.

Bazemore, G. & Griffiths, C. T. (1997). Conferences, circles, boards, and mediations: The new wave of community justice decisionmaking. *Federal Probation*, 61(2), 25-37.

Bazemore, G. & Umbreit, M. (1999). *Conferences, Circles, Boards, and Mediations: Restorative Justice and Citizen Involvement in the Response to Youth Crime*. Washington, DC: Office for Juvenile Justice and Delinquency Prevention (BARJ Project), U.S. Department of Justice.

Clements, C. (1988). Delinquency prevention and treatment: A community centered perspective. *Criminal Justice and Behavior*, pp. 286-305.

Delgado, M. (1996). Puerto Rican food establishments as social service organizations: Results of an asset assessment. *Journal of Community Practice*, pp. 57-77.

Delgado, M. & Santiago, J. (1998). HIV/AIDS in a Puerto Rican/Dominican community: A collaborative project with a botanical shop. *Social Work*, 43, 183-186.

Dembo, R., Shemwell, M., Guida, J., Schmeider, J., Pacheco, K., & Seeberger, W. (1998). A longitudinal study of the impact of a family empowerment on juvenile offender psychological functioning: A first assessment. *Journal of Child & Adolescent Substance Abuse*, 8, 15-54.

Dennis, M. L., Dawud-Noursi, S., Muck, R., & McDermeit, M. (2002). The need for developing and evaluating adolescent treatment models. In S. J. Stevens and A. R.

Morral (Eds.), *Adolescent Substance Abuse Treatment in the United States: Exemplary Models from a National Evaluation Study*. Binghamton, NY: Haworth Press.

Freire, P. (1996). *Pedagogy of the Oppressed*. New York: Labyrinth Books.

Howell, J., Krisberg, B., Hawkins, J., & Wilson, J. (1995). *A Sourcebook: Serious, Violent and Chronic Juvenile Offenders*, Thousand Oaks, CA: Sage Publications.

Lajeunesse, T. & Associates Ltd. (1996). *Evaluation of Community Holistic Circle Healing. Hollow Water First Nation.* Volume 1: Final Report.

Levitt, P. (1995). A todos les llamo primo (I call everyone cousin): The social basis for Latino businesses. In M. Halter (Ed.), *New Immigrants in the Marketplace: Boston's Ethnic Entrepreneurs* (pp. 120-140). Boston: University of Massachusetts Press.

Northwest Frontier Addiction Technology Transfer Center. (2000). *Substance abuse treatment workforce survey: A regional needs assessment.* Prepared by RMC Research Corporation. ix-x, 7, 11-15, 19-20, 22-24.

Pond, A. S., Aguirre-Molina, M., & Orleans, J. (2002). *The adolescent substance abuse treatment workforce: Status, challenges, and strategies to address their particular needs.* Paper prepared for the Robert Wood Johnson Foundation and presented for discussion at the Center for Substance Abuse Treatment's summit on adolescent systems of care (9/26-27/02).

Pranis, K. (2000). Restorative Justice, Social Justice, and the Empowerment of Marginalized Populations. In G. Bazemore and M. Schiff (Eds.), *Restorative Community Justice: Repairing Harm and Transforming Communities.* Cincinnati, OH: Anderson Publishers.

Robbins, M. S., Kumar, S., Walker-Barnes, C., Feaster, D. J., Briones, E., & Szapocznik, J. (2002). Ethnic differences in comorbidity among substance abusing adolescents referred to outpatient therapy. *Journal of the American Academy of Child and Adolescent Psychiatry*, 41(4), 394-401.

Rogler, L., Malgady, R., Costantino, G., & Blumenthal, R. (1987). What do culturally sensitive mental health services mean? The case of Hispanics. *American Psychologist*, pp. 565-570.

Schonberg, S. (1993). *Guidelines for the Treatment of Alcohol and Other Drug-Abusing Adolescents*, Rockville, MD: U.S. Department of Health and Human Services.

Stuart, B. (1996). Circle sentencing in Canada: A partnership of the community and the criminal justice system. *International Journal of Comparative and Applied Criminal Justice*, 20(2).

_____. (1997). *Building Community Justice.*

Szapocznik, J. & Fein, S. (1995). In Jose Szapocznik (Ed.), *A Latino/Latino Family Approach to Substance Abuse Prevention.* Washington, D.C.: Center for Substance Abuse Prevention.

Thornberry, T., Tolnay, S., Flanagan, T., & Glynn, P. (1991). *Children in Custody 1987: A Comparison of Public and Private Juvenile Custody Facilities*, Washington, D.C.: U.S. Department of Justice.

Umbreit, M. S. (2001). *Peacemaking and Spirituality: A Journey Toward Healing & Strength.* St. Paul, MN: Center for Restorative Justice & Peacemaking, University of Minnesota.

Villarruel, F. & Walker, N. (2002), *¿Dónde está la justicia?* Washington, D.C.: Building Blocks for Youth.

Chapter 9

# Alcohol Use Among Adult Puerto Rican Injection Drug Users

Lena M. Lundgren, PhD
LaChelle Capalla, MSW
Linsey Ben-Ami, BA

**SUMMARY.** This study explores the association between race/ethnicity and alcohol use for a population of 27,117 Massachusetts injection drug users. This population had all entered the Massachusetts drug treatment system between 1996-2002. Through logistic regression methods, controlling for age, gender, education, employment and homelessness, the study identified that Puerto Rican IDUs were close to 40% less likely to have ever used alcohol compared to their African American counterparts and 60% less likely to have ever used alcohol compared to their White counterparts. To further verify this finding, a sensitivity analysis was conducted for a subsample (n = 469) of IDUs who were not in treat-

Lena M. Lundgren is Associate Professor at Boston University School of Social Work and Director of the Center on Work and Family, Boston University, 264 Bay State Road, Boston, MA 02215 (E-mail: llundgre@bu.edu).

LaChelle Capalla and Linsey Ben-Ami are Research Assistants at the Center on Work and Family.

The assistance of Deborah Chassler, Senior Research Associate at the Center on Work and Family, is gratefully acknowledged.

[Haworth co-indexing entry note]: "Alcohol Use Among Adult Puerto Rican Injection Drug Users." Lundgren, Lena M., LaChelle Capalla, and Linsey Ben-Ami. Co-published simultaneously in *Alcoholism Treatment Quarterly* (The Haworth Press, Inc.) Vol. 23, No. 2/3, 2005, pp. 149-164; and: *Latinos and Alcohol Use/Abuse Revisited: Advances and Challenges for Prevention and Treatment Programs* (ed: Melvin Delgado) The Haworth Press, Inc., 2005, pp. 149-164. Single or multiple copies of this article are available for a fee from The Haworth Document Delivery Service [1-800-HAWORTH, 9:00 a.m. - 5:00 p.m. (EST). E-mail address: docdelivery@haworthpress.com].

ment and who were interviewed by trained interviewers rather than by administrative intake workers. This sensitivity analysis confirmed the relationship between race/ethnicity and alcohol use for IDUs. This finding suggests that drug treatment for Puerto Rican IDUs should focus on their opiate addiction rather than on poly-drug use. *[Article copies available for a fee from The Haworth Document Delivery Service: 1-800-HAWORTH. E-mail address: <docdelivery@haworthpress.com> Website: <http://www.HaworthPress.com> © 2005 by The Haworth Press, Inc. All rights reserved.]*

**KEYWORDS.** Race, ethnicity, alcohol use, drug use

## *INTRODUCTION*

Overall, the existence of differences in cultural drinking patterns is well documented. In 2002, national studies evidenced significant differences in alcohol use. Of three major racial and ethnic groups (African Americans, Latino, non-Latino Whites), non-Latino Whites report the highest levels of alcohol use and the earliest age of initiating alcohol use. Specifically, in 2002, about 55% of the non-Latino White racial/ethnic group reported alcohol use within the past month while 40% of African Americans and 43% of Latinos also reported alcohol use within the past month. With respect to age, African Americans ages 12-17 were the least likely to report past month alcohol use with a rate of 11%, while the rates for Latino and non-Latino White youths were 17% and 20%, respectively. Among all youth ages 12 to 17, 46% of non-Latino Whites, 45% of Latinos, and 36% of African Americans reported lifetime use of alcohol (SAMSA, Office of Applied Studies, National Survey on Drug Use and Health, 2002).

There were, however, smaller differences between racial/ethnic groups with respect to binge drinking. Among African Americans, the rate for binge alcohol use was 21%, while the rate for non-Latino Whites was 23% and Latinos was 25% (SAMSA, Office of Applied Studies, National Survey on Drug Use and Health, 2002).

Less is known of alcohol use among populations that have histories of long-term drug use. None of the three racial/ethnic groups specified in this study reported alcohol as their primary drug of choice. The African American and non-Latino White subjects reported a slightly higher use of alcohol as their drug of choice in lieu of or in addition to other substances as compared to their Latino counterparts. Latino and non-Latino White women in this sample were significantly more likely to report lifetime use of alcohol as compared to their African American counterparts (Argeriou & Daley, 1997). This study also finds that within the population of chemically dependent, pregnant women, Latinos and non-Latino Whites report using heroin as their drug of choice in higher proportions than their African American counterparts (Argeriou & Daley, 1997).

Among emergency room (ER) patients who report significant substance use, drug use was associated with ethnicity, with non-Latino Whites more likely than African Americans and Latinos to report such use (Cherpitel & Borges, 2002). Among Latinos in this sample, acculturation appears to be significantly associated with drug use. Those scoring high on an acculturation scale were as likely or even more likely than non-Latino Whites to report substance use in the six hours prior to the event warranting an ER visit. The majority of those Latinos high on the acculturation scale reported use of central nervous system depressants/opiates prior to the ER event. Highly acculturated Latinos were also likely to report substance use in the last 12 months with roughly 50% of this sample reporting the use of 2 or more substances, and over one-third reporting use of marijuana (Cherpitel & Borges, 2002). Roughly 21% of this latter sample reported use of stimulants such as cocaine/amphetamines and depressants/opiates. Such drug use behavior suggests similarities between this group of highly acculturated Latinos and non-Latino Whites. Data in this study suggest that substance use among Latinos in the U.S. may have a strong impact on health service utilization. Additional research on gender, ethnicity and acculturation may be necessary to determine the burden of substance use on the ER (Cherpitel & Borges, 2002).

Little comprehensive information is available on racial/ethnic differences in alcohol use among larger samples of long-term drug users. This type of information is critical in order to develop culturally appropriate drug treatment services that respond to cultural differences in poly-drug use. The present study specifically examines whether or not Puerto Rican IDUs, when compared to their non-Latino White and African American counterparts, evidence significant differences in alcohol use. This exploration is conducted for a population of 27,117 injection drug users (IDUs) who all entered the Massachusetts drug treatment system at least once during the years of 1996-2002. These IDUs were actively injecting drugs (they reported having injected drugs in the month prior to treatment entry).

To further test the stability of these findings a sensitivity analysis is conducted where the above relationships between race/ethnicity and alcohol use are examined for a smaller subsample group of injection drug users. This sample of 469 individuals (Puerto Rican, African American and non-Latino White) had all entered drug treatment between 2000-2002 and all reported having injected in the past month. However, unlike the primary sample whom were interviewed by administrative intake workers, this subsample of IDUs were interviewed by trained street outreach workers who conducted the interviews on the street. Further, at the time of the interview the IDUs were not seeking treatment.

## METHODS

The data on patterns of alcohol use in IDUs are examined and compared from two separate studies involving IDUs who all had a history of having entered drug treatment. Logistic regression models developed for this study measure whether the likelihood of ever having used alcohol is associated with race/ethnicity (African American, Puerto Rican, non-Latino White) after controlling for:

1. age,
2. gender,
3. education,
4. employment, and
5. homelessness status

The above relationships were examined for a group of 27,117 individuals who entered drug treatment in Massachusetts at least once during the years 1996-2002 and who reported having injected drugs in the month prior to treatment entry. To further test the stability of these findings, a sensitivity analysis was conducted where the above relationships were examined for a group (n = 469) of injection drug users. This group was comprised of African American, Puerto Rican and non-Latino White IDUs who had entered drug treatment during the same period. The IDUs in this group also reported having injected drugs in the past month. In contrast to the larger population, these IDUs (n = 469) were interviewed by trained street outreach interviewers rather than drug treatment intake administrators. In addition, they were not currently seeking treatment.

## DATA SETS

### MIS (Management Information System) Substance Abuse Treatment Database

Variables originated in an MIS database of all admissions to all substance abuse treatment programs licensed by the Bureau of Substance Abuse Services of the Department of Public Health in the state of Massachusetts for the years 1996-2002. This admissions database was then developed into a client level database that included the drug treatment histories for each individual. This database has been recognized as one of the relatively few state-wide drug treatment databases which is both comprehensive and accurate enough to permit detailed exploration of drug treatment utilization (McCarty, McGuire, Harwood, & Field, 1998). These authors state, "A major strength of the Massachusetts information system is that it is a claims-type database . . ." and therefore ". . . requires complete client data on the admissions record before a claim can be paid" (p. 1097). As a result, there is little missing information in each case file. Data for the primary analysis originate from this database.

### Database Containing Information from In-Person Interviews with 469 IDUs Active in Their Drug Use

Outreach workers in western Massachusetts and in the metro-Boston area of Massachusetts conducted in-person interviews with active adult IDUs. All respondents signed statements of informed consent and were paid a small stipend in appreciation of their participation in the research project. Strict procedures were maintained to protect the confidentiality of participants: respondent names and addresses were not given to the research team; social security numbers, Medicaid numbers and other identifying information of that nature were not collected. Two institutional review boards approved the research protocol. In addition, a Certificate of Confidentiality was obtained from the Substance Abuse and Mental Health Services Administration.

The research team developed the interview questionnaire for the in-person interviews used in this study. It is based partially on the NIDA Risk Behavior Assessment battery. Items that were used from this battery include drug use questions, risk behavior, and demographic information. The questions on psychiatric status and use of mental health services originated from the Addiction Severity Index. Reliability and validity have been established for these measures (Needle et al., 1995; Weatherby, 1994; McLellan, Luborsky, Cacciola, & Griffith, 1985; McLellan, Cacciola, Kushner, Peters, Smith, & Pettinati, 1992; McLellan, Luborsky, O'Brien, & Woody, 1980; Knight et al., 1994).

The interviewers, who also functioned as outreach workers, participated in at least three different one-day training sessions on the use of the research questionnaire, interviewing techniques, administering an informed consent, and tracking and locating respondents.

All respondents were 18 years or older, had injected drugs in the past month, and had utilized a Massachusetts substance abuse treatment facility during the two years prior to the interview. (Treatment was defined as including detoxification, methadone maintenance, outpatient counseling and/or residential treatment. It did not include 12-step programs.)

### Independent Variables

*Race-Ethnicity.* This variable was coded as African American, Puerto Rican and non-Latino White. Identical variables were used in primary and sensitivity analysis. It should be noted that 25% of the treatment sample is Puerto Rican. The population of Latinos who were not Puerto Rican was excluded from this analysis.

*Employment.* Primary analysis: Employment was coded as having ever, for the six years of study, reported being employed, either full- or part-time, at any drug treatment admission. Sensitivity analysis: Employment was coded as whether or not respondent was currently employed, full- or part-time.

*Education.* Primary analysis: Education was recoded as a three-category variable: less than high school, high school graduate, and more than high school, based on information of highest number of years of education reported at last drug treatment entry. Sensitivity analysis: Education was coded as highest level of education reported at the time of interview. The variable was then re-coded into a three-category variable: less than high school, high school graduate, and more than high school.

*Homelessness.* Primary analysis: Homeless status was coded as having ever, for the six years of study, reported being homeless at any treatment admission. Sensitivity analysis: Respondents were asked at time of interview whether or not they were currently homeless.

*Age.* Primary analysis: The variable included is mean age for all treatment episodes. Sensitivity analysis: The age variable is the age reported at the time of the interview.

*Gender.* Primary analysis: Gender was coded as reported at first drug treatment admission. Approximately 72% of the sample were men. Identical variables were used in primary and sensitivity analysis.

### Dependent Variables

The key dependent variable measures whether or not the respondent reports having ever in their lifetime used alcohol. This variable is identical for both primary and sensitivity analysis.

### Statistical Analysis

Binomial logistic regression was used to examine the associations between the independent variables and dependent variables for the two statistical models:

1. Client level analysis of likelihood of having ever used alcohol for IDUs having reported injecting drugs in the past month controlling for race/ethnicity, age, gender, education, employment and homelessness for a population of clients entering drug treatment in Massachusetts, 1996-2002.
2. Client level analysis of likelihood of having ever used alcohol for IDUs having reported injecting drugs in the past month controlling for race/ethnicity, age, gender, education, employment and homelessness for a sample of 469 people who were not in treatment, interviewed by trained interviewers.

### RESULTS

The primary study sample included those IDUs who reported having injected drugs in the past month, who were between the ages of 18 and 75 and who had entered state-licensed drug abuse treatment programs between 1996 and 2002. Hence, only in-depth descriptive information on this population will be discussed further. The ethnic-racial distribution was non-Latino White, 67%; Puerto Rican, 25%; and African American, 8.5% (see Table 1). More than two-thirds were men (72%), and the mean age at treatment admission was 34.6 years (SD = 8.9 years). Average age for initiation of heroin use was 21 (SD = 6.9 years). For the non-Latino White population, average age was 21 years, for African Americans the average age was 20 years, and for Puerto Ricans, the average age was 19 years. It should be noted, however, that there were no significant differences between the different racial/ethnic groups for when they first tried heroin. Just over 35% reported being homeless at the time of any treatment admission. Nearly half were high school

TABLE 1. Univariate Statistics: Massachusetts' IDUs in Drug Treatment 1996-2002, Who Injected Drugs in the Past Month (n = 27,117)

| Variable | Percentage or Mean (SD) |
|---|---|
| **Race/Ethnicity** | |
| Non-Latino White | 66.5% |
| African American | 8.5 |
| Puerto Rican | 25.0 |
| | |
| **Gender** | |
| Women | 28.1% |
| Men | 71.9 |
| | |
| **Mean Age in Years** | 34.6 (8.9) |
| | |
| **Level of Education** | |
| Less than high school | 26.0% |
| High school graduate | 48.5 |
| More than high school | 25.5 |
| | |
| **Homelessness** | |
| Did not report being homeless at time of interview | 64.1% |
| Reported being homeless at time of interview | 35.9 |
| | |
| **Employment** | |
| Did not report being employed | 68.5% |
| Reported being employed | 31.5 |
| | |
| **Alcohol Use** | |
| Reported ever using alcohol | 65.0% |
| Reported using alcohol in the past month | 38.9 |
| Mean age of first alcohol use | 14.0 (3.0) |

graduates with just over one-quarter having less education and one-quarter having more education than high school. Approximately one-third reported that they were employed, full- or part-time, at any treatment admission.

Results in Table 3 show that a larger proportion of non-Latino White and African American IDUs in drug treatment are women compared to Puerto Rican IDUs. For example, 32% of non-Latino White IDUs are women compared to 18% of Puerto Rican IDUs. Puerto Rican IDUs were significantly more likely than the other groups to have less than a high school degree. Also, African American and Puerto Rican IDUs were significantly less likely than non-Latino White IDUs to report employment activity.

TABLE 2. Univariate Statistics: IDUs Who Injected Drugs in the Past Month Prior to Interview, Interviewed by Street Outreach Workers (n = 469)

| Variable | Percentage or Mean (SD) |
|---|---|
| **Race/Ethnicity** | |
| Non-Latino White | 37.5% |
| African American | 37.7 |
| Latino | 24.7 |
| | |
| **Gender** | |
| Women | 27.7% |
| Men | 72.3 |
| | |
| **Mean Age in Years** | 35.96 (10.07) |
| | |
| **Level of Education** | |
| Less than high school | 36.2% |
| High school graduate | 45.8 |
| More than high school | 17.9 |
| | |
| **Homelessness** | |
| Did not report being homeless at time of interview | 56.3% |
| Reported being homeless at time of interview | 43.7 |
| | |
| **Employment** | |
| Did not report being employed | 76.1% |
| Reported being employed | 23.9 |
| | |
| **Alcohol Use** | |
| Reported ever using alcohol | 89.8% |
| Reported using alcohol in the past month (n = 421) | 72.2 |
| Mean age of first alcohol use | 13.75 (3.52) |

TABLE 3. Bivariate Statistics: Massachusetts' IDUs in Drug Treatment 1996-2002, Who Injected Drugs in the Past Month (n = 27,117)

| Variable | Race/Ethnicity | | |
|---|---|---|---|
| | Non-Latino White (n = 18,028) | African American (n = 2,297) | Puerto Rican (n = 6,792) |
| **Gender*** | | | |
| Women | 32.1% | 26.3% | 18.1% |
| Men | 67.9 | 73.7 | 81.9 |
| | | | |
| **Mean Age in Years (SD)** | 34.4 (9.0) | 40.0 (8.2) | 33.2 (8.0) |
| | | | |
| **Education*** | | | |
| Less than high school | 18.3% | 25.8% | 46.6% |
| High school graduate | 50.9 | 51.7 | 41.1 |
| More than high school | 30.8 | 22.5 | 12.4 |
| | | | |
| **Homelessness*** | 35.3% | 38.8% | 36.6% |
| | | | |
| **Employment*** | | | |
| Did not report being employed | 63.3% | 80.4% | 78.0% |
| Reported being employed | 36.7 | 19.6 | 22.0 |
| | | | |
| **Alcohol Use*** | | | |
| Reported ever using alcohol | 68.1% | 66.3% | 56.1% |
| Reported using alcohol in the past month | 39.7 | 48.5 | 33.5 |
| Mean age at first alcohol use (SD) | 13.7 (2.7) | 15.1 (4.2) | 14.6 (3.3) |
| | | | |
| **WOMEN (n = 7,619)** | | | |
| **Alcohol Use*** | | | |
| Have ever used alcohol | 68.1% | 69.9% | 55.6% |
| Used alcohol in the last month | 34.9 | 47.8 | 31.0 |
| Mean age at first alcohol use (SD) | 13.8 (2.9) | 16.2 (5.2) | 15.1 (3.9) |
| | | | |
| **MEN (n = 19,498)** | | | |
| **Alcohol Use*** | | | |
| Have ever used alcohol | 68.2% | 65.0% | 56.2% |
| Used alcohol in the last month (19,498) | 42.0 | 48.7 | 34.0 |
| Mean age at first alcohol use (SD) | 13.6 (2.5) | 14.7 (3.7) | 14.5 (3.1) |

*p = .05
**p = .01
***p = .001

At the bivariate level, Puerto Rican IDUs were significantly less likely to report alcohol use. Only 56% of Puerto Rican IDUs said that they had ever used alcohol when entering treatment compared to approximately 70% of African American and non-Latino White IDUs. How then did this population of IDUs who had entered into the drug treatment system between 1996-2002 differ from a subsample of this population (n = 469) who had entered drug treatment 2000-2002, who were currently active in their drug use, and who were interviewed by trained street outreach workers (Table 2)?

First, as described in Table 4, the IDUs who were identified through street outreach were less educated than the treatment population. For example, 65% of Puerto Rican IDUs identified through street outreach had not completed high school compared to 47% of the Puerto Rican drug treatment population. They were also more likely to be homeless. Interestingly, the Puerto Rican IDU population identified through street outreach did not report, at the bivariate level, statistically significant differences in their alcohol use compared to their African American and non-Latino White counterparts. For each of these three populations of active users, close to 90% reported that they had ever used alcohol. Many more women interviewed by street outreach workers reported having ever used alcohol compared to the women in the drug treatment population (94% of n = 469 compared to 56% of women in the primary sample).

## Results from Logistic Regression

To untangle these relationships identified between race-ethnicity, education, employment, and homelessness, two logistic regression models were developed. As Table 5 describes, for the primary study population, after controlling for gender, age, education, employment and homelessness status, African American and non-Latino White IDUs were significantly more likely to report having ever used alcohol as compared to Puerto Rican IDUs. African Americans were approximately 39% more likely than Puerto Ricans to report having used alcohol. Non-Latino Whites were approximately 64% more likely than Puerto Ricans to report having used alcohol. This finding is consistent with national data on the general population showing that Puerto Rican populations are less likely to use alcohol. The model also identified that women were not significantly less likely than men to use alcohol. Further, those who had more than a high school education were slightly less likely to use alcohol compared to those who had not graduated from high school and

TABLE 4. Bivariate Statistics: IDUs Interviewed by Street Outreach Workers (n = 469)

| Variable | Non-Latino White (n = 177) | African American (n = 176) | Puerto Rican (n = 116) |
|---|---|---|---|
| **Gender** | | | |
| Women | 27.1% | 26.7% | 30.2% |
| Men | 72.9 | 73.3 | 69.8 |
| | | | |
| **Mean Age in Years (SD)*** | 31.9 (10.1) | 39.1 (9.2) | 37.3 (9.3) |
| | | | |
| **Education*** | | | |
| Less than high school | 21.5% | 32.4% | 64.7% |
| High school graduate | 53.7 | 50.6 | 26.7 |
| More than high school | 24.9 | 17.0 | 8.6 |
| | | | |
| **Homelessness*** | | | |
| Reported being homeless | 30.5% | 51.1% | 52.6% |
| Did not report being homeless | 69.5 | 48.9 | 47.4 |
| | | | |
| **Employment*** | | | |
| Employed full or part time or occasionally | 31.6% | 24.4% | 11.2% |
| Unemployed | 68.4 | 75.6 | 88.8 |
| | | | |
| **Alcohol Use** | | | |
| Ever used alcohol | 92.1% | 88.6% | 87.9% |
| Used alcohol in the past month* | 61.0 | 72.2 | 59.5 |
| Mean number of days used alcohol in the past month (SD)*** (n = 304) | 11.4 (9.8) | 16.4 (10.7) | 10.2 (10.6) |
| Mean age of first alcohol use (SD)*** (n = 403) | 12.95 (2.8) | 13.8 (3.4) | 14.8 (4.3) |
| | | | |
| **WOMEN (n = 130)** | | | |
| **Alcohol Use** | | | |
| Ever used alcohol | 81.3% | 78.7% | 94.3% |
| Used alcohol in the past month | 50.0 | 59.6 | 57.1 |
| Mean age first used alcohol (SD)*** (n = 108) | 12.9 (2.5) | 14.7 (3.9) | 17.0 (4.8) |
| Mean number of days used alcohol in the last month (SD) (n = 72) | 12.5 (9.2) | 13.8 (9.3) | 7.9 (10.1) |
| | | | |
| **MEN (n = 339)** | | | |
| **Alcohol Use** | | | |
| Ever used alcohol* | 96.1 | 92.2 | 85.2 |
| Used alcohol in the past month* | 65.1 | 76.7 | 60.5 |
| Mean age of first alcohol use (SD) (n = 295) | 13.0 (2.9) | 13.6 (3.2) | 13.7 (3.7) |
| Mean number of days used alcohol in the last month (SD)*** (n = 232) | 11.0 (10.0) | 17.1 (11.1) | 11.2 (10.8) |

*p = .05
**p = .01
***p = .001

TABLE 5. Logistic Regression: Characteristics Associated with Likelihood of Having Ever Used Alcohol for IDUs in Massachusetts' Drug Treatment (N = 27,117)

| IDU Characteristics | Ever Used Alcohol Odds Ratio (95% CI: Lower, Upper) | |
|---|---|---|
| *Race/Ethnicity* | | |
| Puerto Rican (a) | | |
| Non-Latino White*** | 1.642 | (1.545, 1.746) |
| African American*** | 1.394 | (1.259, 1.543) |
| Women (b) | 1.031 | (.973, 1.092) |
| Age*** | 1.016 | (1.013, 1.019) |
| *Education* | | |
| Less than high school (a) | | |
| High school graduate | .995 | (.922, 1.074) |
| More than high school** | .905 | (.849, .964) |
| Employed (b) | 1.039 | (.982, 1.100) |
| Homeless (b)** | .938 | (.890, .989) |
| Model Chi Square $X^2$ = 452.88, df = 8, p < .001 | | |

(a) Reference group

(b) Yes group is compared to the no group

*p ≤ .05
**p ≤ .01
***p ≤ .001

those who were homeless were slightly less likely to use alcohol compared to those who were not homeless.

To verify the relationship between race/ethnicity and alcohol use described above, a second logistic regression model was developed. This model is described in Table 6. The results from this analysis are generally consistent with the results from the primary analysis. Thus, for the population of 469 IDUs, who were interviewed by trained street outreach interviewers in a non-treatment setting, after controlling for gender, age, education, employment and homelessness, there were still racial/ethnic differences in alcohol use. Specifically, for this population, African Americans were approximately 12% more likely to report having ever used alcohol than Puerto Ricans while non-Latino Whites

TABLE 6. Logistic Regression: Characteristics Associated with Likelihood of Having Ever Used Alcohol for IDUs Interviewed by Street Outreach Workers (N = 469)

| IDU Characteristics | Ever Used Alcohol Odds Ratio (95% CI: Lower, Upper) | |
| --- | --- | --- |
| *Race/Ethnicity* | | |
| Puerto Rican (a) | | |
| Non-Latino White* | 2.442 | (.985, 6.053) |
| African American | 1.121 | (.510, 2.466) |
| Women (b)** | .434 | (.226, .833) |
| Age** | 1.054 | (1.015, 1.095) |
| *Education* | | |
| Less than high school (a) | | |
| High school graduate | .864 | (.290, 2.576) |
| More than high school | .612 | (.221, 1.695) |
| Employed (b) | .665 | (.319, 1.386) |
| Homeless (b) | .825 | (.427, 1.594) |
| Model Chi Square $X^2$ = 19.738, df = 8, * p < .01 | | |

(a) Reference group
(b) Yes group is compared to the no group

* $p \leq .05$
** $p \leq .01$

were more than two and one-half times more likely than Puerto Ricans to report having ever used alcohol. These numbers, especially for the Puerto Rican population, are surprisingly similar for the two groups. Also, similar relationships were identified between age and alcohol for the two groups. For the smaller sample (n = 469), education and homelessness were not statistically significant. In terms of gender, the difference between women as compared to men was significant for the n = 469 sample but not significant in the primary sample (n = 27,117).

## DISCUSSION

Administrative databases, as the one used in the primary analysis of this study, enable researchers to pursue lines of inquiry that would otherwise not be possible. However, these data sets have limitations. For example, such databases tend to include variables that may be less than ideal from a research perspective because the data are obtained by agency-based interviewers whose reliability is unknown. To offset the drawbacks, researchers can enhance the robustness of their results by conducting a sensitivity analysis to demonstrate whether observed relationships hold true under various assumptions.

This study specifically compared the results from one individual level multivariate analysis to another analysis with a subsample of IDUs. The individual level multivariate analysis examined the relationship between race/ethnicity and ever having used alcohol for IDUs who had entered the drug treatment system in 1996-2002. In contrast, the analysis of the IDU subsample examined those who were currently active in their drug use and who were interviewed by trained street outreach worker interviewers. Our results, with respect to the two patterns identified above, were similar for the two groups. This was especially true for the relationships identified between race/ethnicity and alcohol use.

Specifically, the results of this analysis identify that for a population of over 27,000 IDUs having entered the Massachusetts' drug treatment system between 1996-2002, there were significant differences between the alcohol use of Puerto Rican IDUs compared to African American and non-Latino White IDUs. Specifically, Puerto Rican IDUs were close to 40% less likely to report having ever used alcohol compared to their African American counterparts and more than 60% less likely than their non-Latino White counterparts to report having ever used alcohol. This relationship held true even after controlling for factors such as age, gender, education, employment and homelessness.

This relationship between race/ethnicity and alcohol use was also confirmed when examining it in a smaller subsample of IDUs. What does this imply? While the majority of Puerto Rican IDUs do use alcohol, this group as a whole has a significantly lower likelihood to use alcohol, as compared to their non-Latino White counterparts. This suggests that Puerto Rican IDUs are more likely than non-Latino Whites to benefit from treatment which directly responds to their opiate addiction and less likely to need drug treatment which incorporates models for treating alcohol addiction. Second, the study confirms the importance, as suggested by Delgado (1998), of using culturally sensitive intake and screening methods of examining the extent that alcohol use is a problem for an individual seeking treatment for illegal drug use.

### Limitations of Research

Findings should be considered in light of the following limitations:
(1) Only IDUs in Massachusetts were examined. Future research needs
to involve state-by-state comparisons. (2) A limited number of variables
were controlled for. Future studies need to include more complex measures on social capital differences.

## REFERENCES

Argeriou, M., & Daley, M. (1997). An examination of racial and ethnic differences within a sample of Latino, non-Latino White (non-Latino), and African American Medicaid- eligible pregnant substance abusers. *Journal of Substance Abuse Treatment*, 14(5), 489-498.

Cherpitel, C. J., & Borges, G. (2002). Substance use among emergency room patients: An exploratory analysis by ethnicity and acculturation. *American Journal of Drug and Alcohol Abuse*, 28(2), 287-305.

Delgado, M. (1998) *Alcohol Use/Abuse Among Latinos*. Editor. Haworth Press, NY, NY.

Knight, K. R., Holcom, M., & Simpson, D. D. (1994). TCU psychosocial functioning and motivational scales: Manual on Psychometric Properties. Fort Worth, TX: Christian University Institute for Behavioral Research.

McCarty, D., McGuire, T. G., Harwood, H. J., & Field, T. (1998). Using state information systems for drug abuse services research. *American Behavioral Scientist*, 41(8), 1090-1106.

McLellan, A. T., Luborsky, L., O'Brien, C. P., & Woody, G. E. (1980). An improved evaluation instrument for substance abuse patients: The Addiction Severity Index. *Journal of Nervous and Mental Disease*, 168, 26-33.

McLellan, A. T., Luborsky, L., Cacciola, J., & Griffith, J. E. (1985). New data from the Addiction Severity Index: Reliability and validity in three Centers. *Journal of Nervous and Mental Disease*, 173, 412-423.

McLellan, A. T., Cacciola, J., Kushner, H., Peters, F., Smith, I., & Pettinati, H. (1992). The fifth edition of the Addiction Severity Index: Cautions, additions, and normative data. *Journal of Substance Abuse Treatment*, 5, 312-316.

Needle, R. H., Weatherby, N. L., Chitwood, D. D., Booth, R. E., Watters, J. K., Fisher, D. G., Brown, B. S., Cesari, H., Williams, M. L., Andersen, M. D., & Braunstein, M. (1995). Reliability of self-reported HIV risk behaviors of drug users. *Psychology of Addictive Behaviors*, 9(4), 242-250.

Weatherby, N. L., Needle, R. H., Cesari, H., Booth, R. E. et al. (1994). Validity of self-reported drug use among injection drug users and crack cocaine users recruited through street outreach. *Evaluation and Program Planning*, 17(4), 347-355.

Chapter 10

# Substance Abuse Prevention for High-Risk Youth: Exploring Culture and Alcohol and Drug Use

Lori K. Holleran, PhD, ACSW
Margaret A. Taylor-Seehafer, PhD, RN, FNP
Elizabeth C. Pomeroy, PhD, LMSW
James Alan Neff, PhD, MPH

Lori K. Holleran is Assistant Professor, The University of Texas at Austin School of Social Work.

Margaret A. Taylor-Seehafer is Assistant Professor, The University of Texas at Austin School of Nursing.

Elizabeth C. Pomeroy is Associate Professor and BSW Program Director, The University of Texas at Austin School of Social Work.

James Alan Neff is Professor and Director of Research, Department of Psychiatry and Behavioral Sciences, Meharry Medical College.

This study was funded by the Center for Health Promotion and Disease Prevention Research in Underserved Populations (CHPR), The University of Texas at Austin School of Nursing Grant from the National Institute of Nursing Research of the National Institutes of Health. The researchers would like to acknowledge the groundwork provided by the NIDA-funded Drug Resistance Strategies Project (Co-PIS Dr. Flavio Marsiglia and Dr. Michael Hecht).

[Haworth co-indexing entry note]: "Substance Abuse Prevention for High-Risk Youth: Exploring Culture and Alcohol and Drug Use." Holleran, Lori K. et al. Co-published simultaneously in *Alcoholism Treatment Quarterly* (The Haworth Press, Inc.) Vol. 23, No. 2/3, 2005, pp. 165-184; and: *Latinos and Alcohol Use/Abuse Revisited: Advances and Challenges for Prevention and Treatment Programs* (ed: Melvin Delgado) The Haworth Press, Inc., 2005, pp. 165-184. Single or multiple copies of this article are available for a fee from The Haworth Document Delivery Service [1-800-HAWORTH, 9:00 a.m. - 5:00 p.m. (EST). E-mail address: docdelivery@haworthpress.com].

Available online at http://www.haworthpress.com/web/ATQ
doi:10.1300/J020v23n02_10

**SUMMARY.** This pilot study explores issues of culture and alcohol and other drug use in relation to substance abuse prevention with high-risk youth, with a particular interest in Latinos/as and acculturation. Many of the prominent prevention studies are school based, missing some of the youth at very highest risk for alcohol and drug use and abuse. Consequently, this study was conducted in community settings with youth from high-risk neighborhoods and environmental conditions including a homeless youth shelter, an alternative learning setting, and a low-income community program. The data indicated a high lifetime prevalence of drug use (over 80% for Whites and Latinos for beer, wine, liquor, and marijuana), with consistently lower prevalence rates observed among African-Americans. In addition, the study found significant ethnic differences in substance use (last 30 days) in the sample (median age = 16), with African-Americans reporting significantly lower incidence of marijuana and cocaine use ($p < .05$) than other youth. Implications for prevention, intervention and future research are discussed. *[Article copies available for a fee from The Haworth Document Delivery Service: 1-800-HAWORTH. E-mail address: <docdelivery@ haworthpress. com> Website: <http://www.HaworthPress.com> © 2005 by The Haworth Press, Inc. All rights reserved.]*

**KEYWORDS.** Latino youth, acculturation, culture

## *INTRODUCTION*

Growing evidence indicates that culture and environment strongly effect adolescent alcohol and drug beliefs and behaviors (Botvin, Schinke, & Orlandi, 1995). Consequently, while most prevention programs are implemented universally in school settings, often excluding the youth at highest risk for drug use/abuse, this study was conducted in community settings including: (a) a homeless shelter and outreach program for youth in Austin; (b) an alternative learning center for high-risk youth; and (c) a low-income community program for youth. All of the participants were youth from high-risk neighborhoods and adverse environments.

In the United States, few substance abuse prevention approaches have proven effective in reducing substance use among adolescents in general, and even fewer approaches have been evaluated for their effectiveness with ethnic minority youths and youth in high-risk environments (Forgey, Schinke, & Cole, 1997; Gorman, 1998). Most drug prevention programs are created by and for European Americans and tested primarily on this ethnic group. It has been suggested that the failure of many prevention programs can be traced to their lack of cultural sensitivity (Hansen, Miller, & Leukefeld, 1995; Palinkas et al., 1996). Research indicates that tailoring an intervention to a target population can increase its effectiveness (Marsiglia et al., 2000). As a result, there has been a shift to ethnically sensitive programs (Botvin et al., 1995), to enhance program impact (Botvin et al., 1995).

The methodology of this exploratory study included a quantitative survey design to assess cultural issues and substance use patterns as well as qualitative focus groups to gain insight into the youth's perspectives about the role of ethnicity and culture in drug prevention. This project served as a pilot to a larger study that addresses culture, acculturation and drug resistance strategies with multicultural youth in Texas. More specifically, Dr. Holleran conducated this study to launch a series of investigations to be supported through K01 grant [1K01 DA017276-01] from the National Institute on Drug Abuse (NIDA). The aims of the study were to explore ways to assess acculturative types of high-risk youth in community settings, to assess drug use with regard to participant ethnicity and community settings, and to gather qualitative information from the participants related to their sociocultural experience and their perspectives on substances and prevention.

## Literature Review

Recent research on the prevalence of substance abuse in Latino populations shows that the lifetime substance use rates for Latinos are between the higher rates of European Americans and the lower rates of African-Americans (Beauvais & Oetting, 2002); Cuban adolescents have the highest reported 12-month illicit drug use rates of any ethnic group in the U.S. (Wallace et al., 2002). Data from the Monitoring the Future (MTF), a school-based survey, reveal that during the past decade, 8th grade (12 to 13 years old) Latino youth began to display elevated consumption for a variety of substances including alcohol, marijuana, cocaine, heroin, tranquilizers, MDMA (ecstasy), and LSD. Consequently, in the 8th grade, Latinos have the highest rate of substance use for that age group in the nation. However, data from the MTF also indicate that after the 8th grade, prevalence rates of Caucasian substance abuse is comparable to Latinos (Wallace et al., 2002). Among persons 12 years or older in 2001, the rates for illicit drug and alcohol dependence or abuse were 7.8% among Latinos, 7.5% among Whites, and 6.2% among African-Americans (National Household Survey, 2001).

Regarding gender, prevalence data indicate the rate of drug use among Latino females (Latinas) has historically been significantly lower than those of Latino males (Anthony, Warner, & Kessler, 1994; Hughes, Day, Marcantonio, & Torpy, 1997). Latina women report lower rates of substance use compared to non-Latina White women (Young & Harrison, 2001). However, recent studies indicate that Latinas are using at rates increasingly similar to their male counterparts (Warner, Canino, & Colon, 2001), and in some instances higher rates have been reported for females (Kandel, Chen, Warner, Kessler, & Grant, 1997; Sloboda, 2002).

In addition to looking at ethnic cultures, this work purports that the culture of students in traditional education programs varies dramatically from youth in GED programs, low-income community programs, and homeless shelters (Rew, Taylor, & Fitzgerald, 2001). Contextual factors including low SES, lack of school attendance, and absence of family stability have substantial influence on substance use or misuse (Freeman, 2001). The importance of programs for non-school settings is apparent in the high-risk status of adolescents found in these settings. For example, research shows that rates of alcohol and other drug (AOD) use are extremely high among homeless and street youth (Greene, Ennett, & Ringwalt, 1997; Kipke, Montgomery, Simon, & Iverson, 1997; Koopman, Rosario, & Rotheran-Borus, 1994), delinquent youth (Barnes, Welte, & Hoffman, 2002), youth from low SES environments (Eisner, 2002; Epstein, Botvin, & Diaz, 1995; Stewart, 2002), youth with hostile or rejecting parents (Young, Oetting, & Deffenbacher, 1996), violent youth (Elickson, Saner, & McGuigan, 1997), adolescent mothers (Scafidi, Field, & Prodromidis, 1997), and youth with lifestyles oriented around leisure time (Eisner, 2002). In short, youth in non-school settings represent a high-risk group based upon the likelihood of exposure to drugs and drug-using peers as well as likelihood of prior use.

With regard to homeless youth, lifetime rates of alcohol and other drug (AOD) use are higher among homeless and street youth than among sheltered or household youth (Greene et al., 1997). Seventy to eighty percent of street youth report daily use of alcohol, while 35-55% report weekly or greater use of cocaine, crack, heroin, and/or amphetamines (Greene et al., 1997; Kipke, Montgomery, Simon, & Iverson, 1997; Koopman, Rosario, & Rotheran-Borus, 1994).

Examining the overlap of ethnicity and alternative environmental cultures, Koopman and colleagues (1994) report that Hispanic homeless youth are more likely than other ethnic groups (White and Black) to continue use of AOD after leaving home environments. However, a recent study conducted in an urban Texas community did not support this finding (Rew, Taylor, & Fitzgerald, 2001). While the prevalence of AOD use was similar to that reported in other studies of homeless youth, no significant differences were found between White and Hispanic street youth in AOD use at age of onset or use in the past 30 days (Rew, Taylor, & Fitzgerald, 2001). Significantly more research is needed in this area to determine the implications for prevention interventions with high-risk youth.

## Extant Prevention Programs: The Need to Consider Culture and Acculturation

Most well-known substance abuse prevention programs fall into two basic categories: (1) *Information provision models* such as DARE (Becker, Agopian, & Yeh, 1992; Clayton, Leukefeld, Harrington, & Cattarello, 1996; Harmon, 1993; Lynum et al., 1999; Ringwalt, Ennett, & Holt, 1991) and Health Belief Models (Albert & Simpson, 1985), and (2) *Social influence models* including Life Skills Training (Botvin et al., 1990; Botvin, Baker et al., 1995) and the Social Competence Program (Caplan et al., 1992) and Resistance Strategies Training such as Project SMART (Hansen et al., 1988), Project ALERT (Ellickson & Bell, 1990; Ellikson, Bell, & McGuigan, 1993), and DRS (Marsiglia, Kulis, & Hecht, 2000). While the former has generally been found to be ineffective, social influence models have been identified as best practice prevention programs by NIDA and CSAP. Meta-analyses of resistance skills training programs further support their effectiveness (Tobler, 1997).

"Culture," "acculturation," and "ethnicity" have been defined in various ways (Gutmann, 1999), and many studies approach ethnicity in a "glossed" fashion, denying the heterogeneity within groups and other contextual factors (Collins, 1995; Trimble, 1995). Acculturation has often been ignored or oversimplified in prevention efforts (Gutmann, 1999; Koss-Chioino & Vargas, 1999). Historically, the assumption of homogeneity has pervaded the literature obscuring important differences between Mexicans, Cubans, Puerto Ricans, Central Americans, South Americans, Spanish people, and others who have been lumped into the generic "Hispanic" (Felix-Ortiz & Newcomb, 1995). In addition, even when the specific distinction is made, the complexity of acculturative nuances is often overlooked in studies.

As noted, ethnic differences exist with regard to susceptibility to drug use, attitudes regarding drugs, and drug resistance strategies (Collins, 1995; Moon, Hecht, Jackson, & Spellers, 1999). A number of studies document positive relationships between level of acculturation and use of alcohol and other substances (particularly alcohol)–*at least among adults* (Caetano, 1987a, 1987b, 1989; Caetano & Clark, 1998; Caetano & Medina Mora, 1988; Rogler, Cortes, & Malgady, 1991; Felix-Ortiz & Newcomb, 1995). Specifically among *adolescents,* studies have found strong relationships between acculturation and substance abuse (Landrine, Klonoff, & Richardson, 1993), with U.S. born Latino adolescents consistently demonstrating greater ATOD involvement compared with immigrant adolescents (Landrine et al., 1993; Vega & Gil, 1998). In addition, evidence suggests that Latinos who have become highly immersed in dominant culture, particularly females, are at significant risk for substance use and related problems (Caetano & Clark, 2003; Gilbert & Cervantes, 1986; Zapata & Katims, 1994). This is yet another area in need of greater research.

This study began looking at a novel approach in applying the acculturation concept–particularly 'acculturative type'–to the effectiveness of preventive efforts. Acculturation is viewed as encompassing both individual and community level changes produced by the contact between two cultures (Berry, Poortinga, Segall, & Dasen, 1992). Historically, acculturation was viewed as a *linear continuum* from a traditional heritage culture at one end to total assimilation into a dominant host culture at the other (Suarez-Orozco, 2001). It was often oversimplified and measured solely by using language use and length of time in the U.S. as a proxy.

However, in the last 20 years, awareness regarding the complexity of acculturative processes (Caetano & Clark, 2003) and the realization that membership in one group does not preclude membership in another has led to a *multidimensional framework* for understanding acculturation. Noting that (1) people may concurrently immerse in a new culture while maintaining aspects of a heritage culture and (2) individuals may experience detachment from both cultures, Berry (1980) developed a widely cited model of acculturation. Berry conceptualizes four "*acculturative types*" of adaptation: (1) Assimilated (complete adoption of host culture, rejecting heritage culture), (2) integrated (retention of aspects of heritage culture plus adoption of aspects of host culture), (3) separated or segregated (maintenance of heritage culture only) and (4) marginal (abandonment of heritage culture while failing to immerse self in host culture).

This work, in the exploratory stage, aimed to lay the groundwork for future work augmenting extant approaches to tailor intervention content to a specific 'ethnic group' (Berry, 1980; Oetting & Beauvais, 1991). In acknowledging the heterogeneity of ethnic groups, the researchers posit that specific approaches should be more or less effective with regard to individuals in particular acculturative type categories, reflecting the relative orientation to heritage and dominant cultures as well as the amount of acculturative stress experienced.

In order to shift from this linear orientation to the Orthogonal model, inclusion of the Cuellar ARSMA-II measures may offer a vehicle for consideration of the effects of both acculturation *level* and *type*. This pilot utilized this instrument to provide psychometric data on Acculturative Type measures, i.e., Anglo Orientation Scale (AOS) and Mexican Orientation Scale (MOS). Specifically, supplemental analyses allow for use of scores on both AOS and MOS subscales to categorize students as Assimilated, Separated (traditional Mexican), or Integrated (high) Bicultural, which may have a protective effect (see Cuellar et al., 1995 for specific information on this categorization scheme). These supplemental analyses examine differences in substance use and the substance use mediators among students in the different categories, and how transitions between categories influence substance use, mediators of substance use, and the effectiveness of the intervention. Preliminary efforts to construct an acculturation typology involved construction of a linear acculturation score (AOS-MOS) and then standardizing this and applying cut-off points established by Cuellar. While the small sample size limited the meaning of the scores, it is important to begin to utilize these measures and examine the complexity of acculturation with regard to high-risk youth and substance abuse.

## Background and Significance

The Drug Resistance Strategies Project (DRS: R01 DA005629-08) (1997-2001) in Phoenix, Arizona, involved approximately 5,000 Caucasian, Latino/a, and African-American high school youths from large city high schools in the creation of culturally grounded substance abuse prevention videos. The DRS followed from previous research suggesting the utility of *video-based* approaches not only for engaging African-American and Latino youth but also as an effective mode of intervention with these groups (Hecht, Corman, & Miller-Rassulo, 1993; Polansky et al., 1999). The initial DRS project made the important contribution of combining core aspects of social influence models with the added integral component of cultural groundedness. The DRS study findings confirm the theoretical rationale for involvement of minority adolescents in the development of substance abuse prevention projects (Holleran, Reeves, Marsiglia, & Dustman, 2002). The study utilized an experimental design incorporating videos as tools for depicting resistance strategies (Alberts, Miller-Rassulo, & Hecht, 1991; Hecht, Alberts, & Miller-Rassulo, 1992). The videos emphasized values and mores of varied cultures (as identified in preliminary elicitation research with students). For example, while the video depicting Anglo culture portrays individuality, independence from family, and identification with Anglo peers, the Latino video emphasizes familism, ethnic identifications with Latino peers and family, traditional Latino rituals, and language. Analyses of the DRS project data fourteen months post intervention indicated that students in the experimental schools had gained greater confidence in the ability to resist drugs, increased use of the strategies taught by the curriculum to resist substance offers (control schools reported a decrease in the use of these resistance strategies), more conservative norms adopted in both in school and at home, reduction in the use of alcohol (a decrease of nearly 16% in the experimental group and an increase of slightly more than 20% in the control group), and less positive attitudes towards drug use. The most striking implication for the proposed study, however, was that the curricula/videos that integrated elements of minority sociocultural norms were more successful with ethnic minority youth than the Anglo curricula/videos with significant effects on drug norms, attitudes and use, particularly alcohol use. These findings support the importance of culturally grounded information in substance abuse prevention programs. Prevention messages that incorporate cultural elements and are presented within the social context of the participant are more likely to have a positive impact.

This study utilized the student-created videos from the DRS project as a springboard for discussing issues of culture and ethnicity in focus groups. The primary underlying theoretical framework for this study is Contextual Developmental Theory which emphasizes the reciprocity between biological, psychological, social and cultural development in multiethnic youth (Bronfenbrenner, 1995). During adolescence, while youth are undergoing a transitional period of identity and value formation (Erikson, 1950), there are complex interactions between development and cultural context (Harkness & Super, 1983; Koss-Chioino & Vargas, 1999). While there are universal aspects of development such as physical growth, socialization, and shift of referents from adults to peers, these variables interact with culture-specific factors. For example, in a community in which cultural practices include preparing for college, an independent, individuated teenager is not only esteemed, but socially privileged. However, in many Latino cultures where family is a central value, teenagers may opt to stay at home to care for younger siblings. While they are esteemed for this choice within their culture, they may be viewed by the dominant culture as disadvantaged or socially handicapped in terms of educational goals. Thus, culture cannot simply be viewed as an independent variable–it must be viewed as an integral, complex, dynamic aspect of development (Bronfenbrenner, 1995; Valsiner, 1989).

## *Methodology*

This exploratory pilot involved 72 adolescents (33 boys; 37 girls) drawn from community-based programs in Austin, Texas. In addition to the specific aims noted earlier, this pilot study served to: (1) build solid foundations with the community sites, (2) provide preliminary data on substance abuse prevalence among adolescents (and ethnic differences in drug usage), and (3) begin to provide psychometric data on Cuellar's Acculturative Type measures (Anglo Orientation Scale [AOS] and Mexican Orientation Scale [MOS]) among Anglo, Mexican- American, and African-American youth. Pilot data demonstrate the feasibility of recruitment and measurement strategies for a larger implementation of the drug resistance strategies program in these settings.

Participants for the study consisted of adolescents between the ages of 13 and 17 who were involved in one of three programs: the homeless and outreach program of Lifeworks, Inc., the alternative learning center and an East Austin low-income community center (Boys and Girls Club). The agencies involved in the study distributed and collected consent forms prior to the day of research at each agency. More than one sibling from a family was permitted to participate in the study. Adolescents who chose not to participate in the study were still given the opportunity to view the video.

Demographics of the respondents were as follows:

| Variable | % (N) |
|---|---|
| Site | |
| Shelter | 22% (16) |
| Boys/Girls Club | 42% (30) |
| Alternative School | 36% (26) |
| Ethnicity | |
| White | 15% (11) |
| African-American | 53% (38) |
| Hispanic/Latino | 32% (23) |
| Age (mean: range) | 15.3 (11-24) |

To examine the research questions, three groups were established–
one at each location. Participants in the group self-selected from the total number of agency participants. A pre-experimental group design using a survey format was utilized with each group of participants. In
addition, a focus group was conducted with participants following the
video to gain additional information about the impact of the video, their
perceptions and sociocultural relatedness to the adolescents depicted in
the video.

Procedurally, once consent and assent were obtained, researchers explained the study with agency mentors present. An initial survey was
given to the youth to ascertain demographic information and baseline
information about the youth's attitudes and behaviors with regard to
drugs and alcohol using questions adapted from Texas Commission on
Alcohol and Drug Abuse (2000). Measurement of *acculturation level*
was based on the updated Acculturation Rating Scale for Mexican
Americans (ARSMA-II) (Cuéllar & Arnold, 1995). The ARSMA-II
consists of two subscales, a 17-item Mexican Orientation subscale
(MOS) and a 13-item Anglo Orientation subscale (AOS), with all items
responded to on a scale of 1 = "Not at all" to 5 = "Extremely often or almost always." The scales requested information about language use and
preference, ethnic identity and classification, cultural heritage and ethnic behaviors, and ethnic interaction.

Second, two videos were shown: "The Ride" (non-Latino) and "The
Fiesta" (Latino). Third, surveys were distributed to the youth in order to
measure (1) frequencies of resistance strategy usage and (2) responses
to the videos. Responses to the videos were tested using the Perception
of Performance Scale (Miller, Hecht, & Stiff, 1998) developed and utilized with youths in Arizona. With regard to the videos, the Likert scales
address three dependent variables: interest, realism/believability, and

identification with video characters and language. Fourth, following the survey, audio-taped focus groups were used to obtain feedback on their reactions to the videos and again assess the resistance strategies utilized by the Texas youths. Focus groups (Edmunds, 1999) were conducted and will be reported on in a future manuscript. The youth were all invited to discuss the videos along with agency mentors. Focus groups were limited to 30 minutes in order to consider the limited agency time allotted and participants' attention spans.

## Quantitative Data Analysis and Findings

Data gathered included demographic information and substance related information as noted above. In addition to substance use data, the reactions to the videos (e.g., interest, realism/believability, and identification with video characters and language) were added as test variables. Ethnicity and gender were also examined in posthoc analysis of the data if a significant difference between groups was found.

Acculturation, as noted earlier, was measured with the ARSMA-II Revised. This scale was used in two ways. First, the mean of the MOS items was subtracted from the mean of the AOS items to produce a linear acculturation score. This score assesses acculturation along a continuum from very Mexican oriented to very Anglo (or mainstream) oriented. This score demonstrated a test-retest reliability of .96 over one week, and alphas of .88 and .83 for the MOS and AOS subscales, respectively.

Analyses indicated a high lifetime prevalence of drug use (over 80% for Whites and Latinos for beer, wine, liquor, and marijuana), with consistently lower prevalence rates observed among African-Americans. These data indicate the high-risk nature of this population, emphasizing the need for tertiary prevention efforts.

### Lifetime Prevalence of Drug Use

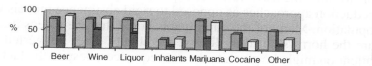

Analyses also indicated significant ethnic differences in substance use (last 30 days) in the sample (median age = 16), with African-Americans reporting significantly lower incidence of marijuana and cocaine use (p < .05) compared to other youth.

Prevalence (Last 30 Days) of Drug Use

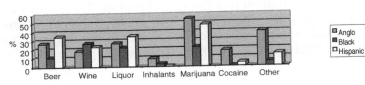

Further psychometric analyses examined: (1) the internal consistency reliability of AOS and MOS dimensions among ethnic subgroups of youth, and (2) whether AOS and MOS composite scores would differ among Anglo, African-American, and Hispanic youth.

### *Qualitative Findings*

The youth in all three settings consistently reported that the Latino video was "more realistic," and truer to "real world situations." They found the video to be "more interesting" and noted that they identified more strongly with it than the Anglo video. It is important to note, however, that the two videos are not designed similarly and that the music, script, characters, pace, and style of the videos are in no way parallel for clear comparisons. The students commented that the Anglo video seemed "outdated" and "boring," in contrast with the Latino video, which they described as "interesting" and "cool."

At the homeless youth shelter, during the focus group, participants were articulate, energetic, and interactive. They offered feedback, which often included anecdotes about their own use and the plight of their using peers. One adolescent Anglo female reported that she is helping a friend to cut down on heroin and encouraging her to "only use pot and alcohol" to "kick the hard stuff." This points towards a consideration of harm reduction approaches as opposed to rigid abstinence models with this population. Many of the participants noted that the videos did not "capture the horrors" of drug life on the streets. They suggested that more attention might be given to the consequences, despite the fact that historically, "scare tactics" have not been very effective in prevention (DeJong, 2000). They got excited at the prospect of someday creating their own drug prevention videos. In addition, they noted that "getting high" is a way to survive and cope on the streets and that it is the norm. Several of the participants shared that it is unlikely that anyone in their culture would pressure another to use because "that would leave less drugs for them." One of the shelter counselors poignantly commented, "Most of our kids get high. Some of them are high right now. We only really get a chance to intervene with the worst cases."

At the community center site, the milieu was more cohesive and the participants were very connected with each other and the agency staff. They were relatively uninterested in the Anglo video except for some laughter at parts that they criticized as "stupid" (e.g., when the characters are afraid to be in the care with the girls who are getting high), but the Latino video prompted the participants' interest and they actually sang along with a popular song that ran at the end, during the credits. The feedback revolved around their belief that the videos need to have more "realistic" situations. While they had a difficult time articulating the specific situations, it seemed that they did not feel that the videos accurately depicted their own pressures, drug offers, and life experiences.

Finally, in the Alternative Learning School, where most of the participants were Latino/a and pursuing their GEDs, the students watched the videos attentively. They responded with concern, saying that prevention interventions must capture the "truth" about drugs. Several participants said that many of them choose to use substances and do not have what they consider "serious consequences." The participants suggested that they feel it would impact them more to hear "kids like us" talking about their life experiences and thought that testimonies would impact them more than acted out videos. The teachers in the school also conveyed that this is a "major issue" for their students and that many of their students come to school under the influence of substances, even regularly.

## Study Limitations

Preliminary efforts to construct an acculturation typology involved construction of a linear acculturation score (AOS-MOS) and then standardizing this and applying cut-off points established by Cuellar. The results indicated that the sample was rather mixed in terms of acculturation: 16% of the sample fell in the "predominantly Mexican" category, 17% fell in the "somewhat Mexican" category, approximately 58% fell in the "somewhat Anglo" category, and very few (approximately 9%) fell in the "predominantly Anglo" category. However, as noted, the use of this tool can only be viable with a larger sample.

While the findings show lower prevalence rates among the African-American youth, consistent with the literature, one must consider the fact that the African-American youth in this study were likely at lower risk than the other youth due to the presence of family, community, and school supports when compared to the street youth (predominantly Anglo) and the youth in the alternative learning school (predominantly Latino).

Since the data relied on the Austin area sample, findings cannot be generalized to other locales. The findings of this study are further limited given its exploratory nature. Descriptive data will be utilized to further develop the testing instrument and research design for future quasi-experimental and experimental studies. The researchers intend to refine and develop a drug resistance strategies intervention for adolescent youth use based on the findings from this study.

## DISCUSSION

In some ways, it is a misnomer to consider potential interventions with this population "prevention" considering the high lifetime prevalence of substance use of the youth in this study (i.e., over 80% of the Anglo and Latino youth have used alcohol and marijuana). Attempts to influence knowledge, attitudes, and behaviors of this high-risk population would be considered tertiary prevention at best.

As noted, the youth found the Latino video clearly more resonant culturally than the Anglo video. This may be a function of some of the difficulties in the design and production of the videos (see Holleran et al., 2002) including (1) how difficult it is to capture a quintessential "White culture," (2) the rapidly changing and regionally specific nature of "pop culture" (e.g., popular music, clothing, current language), and (3) the differences between the culture and scenarios of the population targeted with the DRS videos (i.e., universal targeting in junior high schools) and the high-risk population of the youth in this study. Ultimately, interventions must be designed as culturally grounded for the high-risk populations and settings being targeted. It is critical to involve adolescents in the research, intervention designs, and implementation of prevention programs.

While the pilot sample in this exploratory study is too small for definitive analyses, the data do support several important points: (1) adolescents in non-school settings will participate in research activities; (2) adolescents in these settings are ethnically heterogeneous; (3) respondents are willing to report high levels of substance abuse; (4) high reported prevalence of substance abuse supports the high-risk nature of the population; and (5) Cuellar's acculturation measure appears to be promising regarding reliability in different ethnic groups and serves to differentiate among Anglos, African-Americans, and Latinos. More research is needed to explore issues of acculturation, ethnicity, and substance abuse in high-risk youth, particularly in non-school settings.

In order to provide the foundation for further and more expansive research in the area of acculturative type and substance abuse, several implications are clear. First, it is critical that a variety of community-based settings with diverse youth be studied (e.g., community centers, wellness clinics, shelters, alternative schools, and other youth agencies such as drop-in centers for GLBT youth, etc.). Comparison groups should be used in the research wherever feasible. Qualitative and quantitative data should be examined. Concept definitions should be clear and wherever possible, complex issues (e.g., ethnicity, acculturation) should not be oversimplified. Ethnography and other naturalistic research is recommended in order to have the youth and other key informants involved in defining their own culture, motivations, influences with regard to substance abuse research and prevention interventions.

## REFERENCES

Aktan, G.B. (1999). Evolution of a substance abuse prevention program with inner-city African American families. *Drugs & Society, 12*(1/2), 39-52.

Alberts, J.K., Miller-Rassulo, & Hecht, M.L. (1991). A typology of drug resistance strategies. *Journal of Applied Communication Research, 19*, 129-151.

Alberts, W.G. & Simpson, R.I. (1985). Evaluating an educational program for the prevention of impaired driving among grade school students. *Journal of Drug Education, 15*, 57-71.

Anthony, J.C., Warner, L.A., & Kessler, R.C. (1994). Comparative epidemiology of dependence on tobacco, alcohol, controlled substances, and inhalants: Basic findings from the National Comorbidity Survey. *Experimental and Clinical Pyschopharmacology, 2*(3), 244-268.

Barnes, G.M., Welte, J.W., & Hoffman, J.H. (2002). Relationship of alcohol use to delinquency and illicit drug use in adolescents: Gender, age, and racial/ethnic differences. *Journal of Drug Issues, 32*(1), 153-178.

Beauvais, F. & Oetting, E.R. (2002). Variances in the etiology of drug use among ethnic groups of adolescents. *Public Health Report, 117*(1), S8-S14.

Becker, H.K., Agopian, M.W., & Yeh, S. (1992). Impact evaluation of drug abuse resistance education (DARE). *Journal of Drug Education, 22*, 283-292.

Berry, J.W. (1980). Acculturation as varieties of adaptation. In A.M. Padilla (Ed.), *Acculturation: Theory, Models and Some New Findings* (pp. 9-25). Boulder, CO: Westview.

Berry, J.W., Poortinga, Y.H., Segall, M.H., & Dasen, P.R. (1992). *Cross-Cultural Psychology: Research and Applications*. New York: Cambridge University Press.

Botvin, G.J., Baker, E., & Dusenbury, L. (1995). Long-term followup results of a randomized drug abuse prevention trial in a white middle class population. *Journal of the American Medical Association, 273*(14), 1106-1112.

Botvin, G.J., Baker, E., Dusenbury, L., Tortu, S., & Botvin, E.M. (1990). Preventing adolescent drug abuse through a multimodal cognitive-behavioral approach: Results of a 3-year study. *Journal of Consulting and Clinical Psychology, 58*(4), 437-446.

Botvin, G.J., Baker, E., Filazzola, A., & Botvin, E.M. (1990). A cognitive-behavioral approach to substance abuse prevention: A 1-year followup. *Addictive Behavior, 15*, 47-65.

Botvin, G.J., Schinke, S., & Orlandi, M.A. (1995). *Drug Abuse Prevention with Multiethnic Youth*. Sage: Thousand Oaks, London, New Delhi.

Botvin, G.J., Schinke, S.P., Epstein, J.A., & Diaz, T. et al. (1995). Effectiveness of culturally focused and generic skills training approaches to alcohol and drug abuse prevention among minority adolescents: Two-year followup results. *Psychology of Addictive Behaviors, 9*, 183-194.

Bronfenbrenner, U. (1995). Developmental ecology through space and time: A future perspective. In P. Moen, G.H. Elder, & K. Luscher (Eds.), *Examining Lives in Context: Perspectives on the Ecology of Human Development*. Washington, DC: American Psychological Association.

Caetano, R. & Clark, C.L. (1998). Trends in drinking patterns among Whites, Blacks and Hispanics: 1984-1995. *Journal of Studies on Alcohol, 59*, 659-668.

Caetano, R. & Clark, C.L. (2003). Acculturation, alcohol consumption, smoking, and drug use among Hispanics. In K.M. Chun, P.B. Organista, & G. Marin (Eds.), *Acculturation: Advances in Theory, Measurement, and Applied Research*, 223-239. Washington, DC: American Psychological Association.

Caetano, R. & Medina Mora, M.E. (1988). Acculturation and drinking among people of Mexican decent in Mexico and the United States. *Journal of Studies on Alcohol, 49*, 462-471.

Caetano, R. (1987a). Acculturation and drinking patterns among U.S. Hispanics. *British Journal of Addiction, 82*, 789-799.

Caetano, R. (1987b). Acculturation, drinking and social setting among U.S. Hispanics. *Drug and Alcohol Dependence, 19*, 215-226.

Caetano, R. (1989). Differences in alcohol use between Mexican Americans in Texas and California. *Hispanic Journal of Behavioral Sciences, 11*, 58-69.

Caplan, M., Weissberg, R.P., Grober, J.S., Sivo, P.J., Grady, K., & Jacoby, C. (1992). Social competence promotion with inner-city and suburban young adolescents: Effects on social adjustment and alcohol use. *Journal of Consulting and Clinical Psychology, 60*, 56-63.

Cherry, V.R., Belgrave, F.Z., Jones, W., Kennon, D.K., Gray, F.S., & Phillips, F. (1998). NTU: An Africentric approach to substance abuse prevention among African American youth. *The Journal of Primary Prevention, 18*(3), 319-339.

Chun, K.M., Organista, P.B., & Marin, G. (2003). *Acculturation: Advances in Theory, Measurement, and Applied Research.* Washington, DC: American Psychological Association.

Clayton, R.R., Leukefeld, C.G., Harrington, N.G., & Cattarello, A. (1996). DARE Drug Abuse Resistance Education: Very popular but not very effective (pp. 101-109). In C.B. McCoy, L.R. Metsch, & J.A. Inciardi (Eds.), *Intervening with Drug-Involved Youth.* Thousand Oaks, CA: Sage Publications.

Collins, R.L. (1995). Issues of ethnicity in research on prevention of substance abuse. In G.J. Botvin, S. Schinke, & M.A. Orlandi (Eds.), *Drug Abuse Prevention with Multiethnic Youth.* Sage: Thousand Oaks, London, New Delhi.

Cuellar, I. & Arnold, B. (1995). Acculturation Rating Scale for Mexican Americans-II: A revision of the original ARSMA scale. *Hispanic Journal of Behavioral Sciences, 17*(3), 275-305.

DeJong, W. (2000). Scare Tactics. Prevention Pipeline, accessed on January 13, 2004. *http://www.edc.org/hec/pubs/articles/scare-tactics.html.*

Edmunds, H. (1999). *The Focus Group Research Handbook.* Thousand Oaks, CA: Sage.

Eisner, M. (2002). Crime, problem drinking, and drug use: Patterns of problem behaviors in cross-national perspective. *The Annals of the American Academy of Political and Social Science, 580,* 201-225.

Elickson, P., Saner, H., & McGuigan, K.A (1997). Profiles of violent youth: substance use and other concurrent problems. *American Journal of Public Health, 87,* 985-991.

Ellickson, P.L. & Bell, R.M. (1990). Drug prevention in junior high: A multi-site longitudinal test. *Science, 247,* 1299-1305.

Ellickson, P.L., Bell, R.M., & McGuigan, K. (1993). Preventing adolescent drug use: Long-term results of a junior high program. *American Journal of Public Health, 83*(6), 856-861.

Epstein, J.A., Botvin, G.J., Diaz, T., Toth, V., & Schinke, S.P. (1995). Social and personal factors in marijuana use and intentions to use drugs among inner city minority youth. *Journal of Developmental and Behavioral Pediatrics, 16,* 14-20.

Epstein, J.A., Botvin, G.J., & Diaz, T. (1995). The role of social factors and individual characteristics in promoting alcohol use among inner-city minority youth. *Journal of Studies on Alcohol, 56,* 39-46.

Erikson, E.H. (1950). *Childhood and Society.* New York: Norton.

Felix-Ortiz, M. & Newcomb, M.D. (1995). Cultural identity and drug use among Latino and Latina adolescents. In G.J. Botvin, S. Schinke, & M.A. Orlandi (Eds.), *Drug Abuse Prevention with Multiethnic Youth* (pp. 147-165). Thousand Oaks, CA: Sage.

Forgey, M.A., Schinke, S., & Cole, K. (1997). School-based interventions to prevent substance use among inner-city minority adolescents. In D.K. Willson, J.R. Rodrigue, & W.C. Taylor (Eds.), *Health-Promoting and Health-Compromising Behaviors Among Minority Adolescents.* Washington, D.C.: American Psychological Association.

Freeman, E.M. (2001). *Substance Abuse Intervention, Prevention, Rehabilitation, and Systems Change Strategies: Helping Individuals, Families, and Groups to Empower Themselves.* New York: Columbia University Press.

Gilbert, M.J. & Cervantes, R.C. (1986). Patterns and practices of alcohol use among Mexican-Americans: A comprehensive review. *Hispanic Journal of Behavioral Sciences, 8,* 1-60.

Gorman, D.M. (1998). The irrelevance of evidence in the development of school-based drug prevention policy, 1986-1996. *Evaluation Review, 22,* 118-146.

Greene, J.M., Ennett, S.T., & Ringwalt, C.L. (1997). Substance use among runaway and homeless youth in three samples. *American Journal of Public Health, 87,* 229-235.

Gutmann, M.C. (1999). Ethnicity, alcohol, and acculturation. *Social Science and Medicine, 48,* 173-184.

Hansen, W.B., Johnson, C.A., Flay, B.R., Graham, J.W., & Sobel (1988). Affective and social influence approaches to the prevention of multiple substance abuse among seventh grade students: Results from Project SMART. *Preventive Medicine, 17,* 135-154.

Hansen, W.B., Miller, T.W., & Leukefeld, C.G. (1995). Prevention research recommendations: Scientific integration for the 90's. *Drugs & Society, 8*(3/4), 161-167.

Harkness, S. & Super, C.M. (1983). The cultural construction of child development: A framework for the socialization of affect. *Ethos 11*(4), 221-231.

Harmon, M.A. (1993). Reducing the risk of drug involvement among early adolescents: An evaluation of drug abuse resistance education (DARE). *Evaluation Review, 17,* 221-239.

Hecht, M.L., Alberts, J.K., & Miller-Rassulo, M. (1992). Resistance to drug offers among college students. *International Journal of the Addictions, 27,* 995-1017.

Hecht, M.L., Corman, S., & Miller-Rassulo, M. (1993). An evaluation of the drug resistance project: A comparison of film versus live performance. *Health Communication, 5,* 75-88.

Hecht, M.L., Trost, M., Bator, R., & McKinnon, D. (1997). Ethnicity and gender similarities and difference in drug resistance. *Journal of Applied Communication Research, 25,* 75-97.

Holleran, L., Reeves, L., Marsiglia, F.F., & Dustman, P. (2002) Creating culturally-grounded videos for substance abuse prevention: A dual perspective on process. *Journal of Social Work Practice in the Addictions.*

Hughes, T.L., Day, L.E., Marcantonio, R.J., & Torpy, E. (1997). Gender differences in alcohol and other drug use among young adults. *Substance Use & Misuse, 32*(3), 317-342.

Kipke, M.D., Montgomery, S.B., Simon, R.R., & Iverson, E.F. (1997). Substance abuse disorders among runaway and homeless youth. *Substance Use and Misuse, 32,* 965-982.

Klonoff, E.A. & Landrine, H. (1999). Acculturation and alcohol use among Blacks: The benefits of remaining culturally traditional. *The Western Journal of Black Studies, 23*(4), 211-216.

Koopman, C., Rosario, M., & Rotheram-Borus, M.J. (1994). Alcohol and drug use and sexual behaviors placing runaways at risk for HIV infection. *Addictive Behaviors, 19,* 95-103.

Koss-Chioino, J.D. & Vargas, L.A. (1999). *Working with Latino Youth: Culture, Development, and Context.* San Francisco: Jossey-Bass.

Lambert, W.E. & Taylor, D.M. (1990). *Coping with Cultural and Racial Diversity in Urban America.* New York: Praeger.

Landrine, H. & Klonoff, E.A. (1996). *African-American Acculturation: Deconstructing Race and Reviving Culture.* Thousand Oaks, CA, London, & New Delhi: Sage Publications, Inc.

Landrine, H., Klonoff, E.A., & Richardson, J.L. (1993). *Cultural diversity in the predictors of adolescent substance use.* Paper presented at the annual meeting of the Association for Advancement of Behavior Therapy, Atlanta, GA.

Lynum, D.R., Milich, R., Zimmerman, R., Novack, S.P., Logan, T.K., Martin, C., Leukefeld, C., & Clayton, R. (1999). Project DARE: No effects at 10 year follow-up. *Journal of Consulting and Clinical Psychology, 67*(4), 590-593.

Marsiglia, F.F., Kulis, S., & Hecht, M.L. (2000). *Drug Resistance Strategies: The Next Generation.* (NIH/NIDA No. RFA-DA-01-009, The Next Generation of Drug Abuse Prevention Research). Tempe, AZ: Arizona State University. Drug Resistance Strategies Project.

Miller, M., Hecht, M., & Stiff, J. (1998). A exploratory measurement of engagement with live and film media. *Journal of the Illinois Speech and Theatre Association, 49,* 69-86.

Moon, D.G., Hecht, M.L., Jackson, K.M., & Spellers, R. (1999). Ethnic and gender differences and similarities in adolescent drug use and the drug resistance process. *Substance Use and Misuse, 34,* 1059-1083.

Moore, S.E. (2001). Substance abuse treatment with adolescent African American males: Reality therapy with an Afrocentric approach. *Journal of Social Work Practice in the Addictions, 1*(2), 21-32.

National Institute on Drug Abuse (NIDA) (1997-2001). *Drug Resistance Strategies Project* (project number 2RO1 DA05629). Washington, DC: NIH.

Nobles, W.W. (1986). *African Psychology.* Oakland, CA: Blake Family Institute.

Oetting, E.R. & Beauvais, F. (1990-91). Orthogonal cultural identification theory: The cultural Acculturation Status on Delinquency for Mexican-American Adolescents. *American Journal of Community Psychology, 27*(2), 189-211.

O'Malley, P.M., Bachman, J.G., & Johnston, L.D. (1983). Reliability and consistency in self-reports of drug use. *The International Journal of the Addictions, 18,* 806-824.

Palinkas, L.A., Atkins, C.J., Jerreira, D., & Miller, C. (1996). Effectiveness of social skills training form primary and secondary prevention of drug use in high-risk female adolescents. *Preventive Medicine 25,* 692-701.

Polansky, J.M., Buki, L.P., Horan, J.J., Ceperich, S.D., & Burows, D.D. (1999). The effectiveness of substance abuse prevention videotapes with Mexican-American adolescents. *Hispanic Journal of Behavioral Sciences, 21*(2), 186-198.

Ringwalt, C., Ennett, S.T., & Holt, K.D. (1991). An outcome evaluation of project DARE (drug abuse resistance education). *Health Education Research, 6,* 327-337.

Rogler, L.H., Cortes, D.E., & Malgady, R.G. (1991). Acculturation and mental health status among Hispanics: Convergence and new directions for research. *American Psychologist, 46,* 585-597.

Scafidi, F.A., Field, T., & Prodromidis, M. (1997) Psychosocial stressors of drug-abusing disadvantaged adolescent mothers. *Adolescence, 32,* 93-100.

Sloboda, Z. (2002). Changing patterns of "drug abuse" in the United States: Connecting findings from macro- and microepidemiologic studies. *Substance Use & Misuse, 37,* 1229-1251.

Suarez-Orozco, M. (2001). Everything you ever wanted to know about assimilation but were afraid to ask. In R. Hunt (Ed.), *Personalities and Cultures* (pp. 56-78). New York: Natural History Press.

Szapocznik, J. & Kurtines, W. (1993). Family psychology and cultural diversity. *Hispanic Journal of Behavioral Sciences, 48,* 400-407.

Texas Commission on Alcohol and Drug Abuse (2000). 1998 Texas school survey of substance use among students on the border: Grades 4-12. TCADA.

Tobler, N.S. & Stratton, H.H. (1997) Effectiveness of school-based drug prevention programs: A meta-analysis of the research. *Journal of Primary Prevention, 18*(1), 71-128.

Trimble (1995). Toward an understanding of ethnicity and ethnic identity, and their relationship with drug use research. In G.J. Botvin, S. Schinke, & M.A. Orlandi (Eds.), *Drug Abuse Prevention with Multiethnic Youth* (pp. 28-45). Thousand Oaks, CA: Sage.

Valsiner, J. (1989). *Human Development and Culture.* Lexington, MA: Heath.

Vega, W.A. & Gil, A.C. (1999). A model for explaining drug use behavior among Hispanic adolescents. *Drugs and Society, 14*(1-2), 57-74.

Vega, W.A., Gil, A.G., & Wagner, E. (1998). Cultural adjustment and Hispanic adolescent drug use. In W.A. Vega & A.G. Gil (Eds.), *Drug Use and Ethnicity in Early Adolescence* (pp. 125-148). New York: Plenum Press.

Wallace, J.M., Bachman, J.G., O'Malley, P.M., Johnston, L.D., Schulenberg, J., & Cooper, S.M. (2002). Tobacco, alcohol, and illicit drug use: Racial and ethnic differences among U.S. high school seniors, 1976-2000. *Public Health Report, 117,* S67-S75.

Young, S.L., Oetting, E.R., & Deffenbacher, J.L. (1996) Correlations among maternal rejection, dropping out of school, and drug use in adolescents: A pilot study. *Journal of Clinical Psychology, 52,* 96-102.

Young, V.D. & Harrison, R. (2001). Race/ethnic differences in the sequences of drugs used by women. *Journal of Drug Issues, 31*(2), 293-324.

Zapata, J.T. & Kaims, D.S. (1994). Antecedents of substance use among Mexican-American school-age children. *Journal of Drug Education, 24*(3), 233-251.

Chapter 11

# Pentecostal Religion, Asset Assessment and Alcohol and Other Drug Abuse: A Case Study of a Puerto Rican Community in Massachusetts

Melvin Delgado, PhD
Michael Rosati, MA

**SUMMARY.** Religious support systems offer much promise for collaborative interventions with alcohol and other drug abuse organizations. This article presents a case study of an asset assessment of eleven Puerto Rican Pentecostal churches in a New England community and the alcohol and other drug abuse and other types of services provided to the community. A set of recommendations will be presented for the development

---

Melvin Delgado is Professor of Social Work and Chair of Macro Practice Sequence, Boston University School of Social Work, 264 Bay State Road, Boston, MA 02215.

Michael Rosati is affiliated with the Education Development Center, 55 Chapel Street, Newton, MA 02160.

The authors wish to acknowledge the work of Ms. Carmen Cordero, research assistant, and the ministers without whom this manuscript would not be possible.

The research that this article is based upon was funded through a demonstration grant from the Center for Substance Abuse Prevention (5 H86 SP02208), Rockville, MD.

[Haworth co-indexing entry note]: "Pentecostal Religion, Asset Assessment and Alcohol and Other Drug Abuse: A Case Study of a Puerto Rican Community in Massachusetts." Delgado, Melvin, and Michael Rosati. Co-published simultaneously in *Alcoholism Treatment Quarterly* (The Haworth Press, Inc.) Vol. 23, No. 2/3, 2005, pp. 185-203; and: *Latinos and Alcohol Use/Abuse Revisited: Advances and Challenges for Prevention and Treatment Programs* (ed: Melvin Delgado) The Haworth Press, Inc., 2005, pp. 185-203. Single or multiple copies of this article are available for a fee from The Haworth Document Delivery Service [1-800-HAWORTH, 9:00 a.m. - 5:00 p.m. (EST). E-mail address: docdelivery@haworthpress.com].

Available online at http://www.haworthpress.com/web/ATQ
doi:10.1300/J020v23n02_11

of agency collaborative projects/activity with this important Puerto Rican natural support system. *[Article copies available for a fee from The Haworth Document Delivery Service: 1-800-HAWORTH. E-mail address: <docdelivery@haworthpress.com> Website: <http://www.HaworthPress.com>*

**KEYWORDS.** Puerto Ricans, Pentecostals, services, natural supports

## *INTRODUCTION*

Indigenous community resources such as religious support systems offer much promise for collaborative interventions with alcohol and other drug abuse organizations and probably nowhere is this more needed than when addressing the needs of communities of color within the United States. Religious support systems take on even greater prominence in communities where the primary language used is not English and the members of these communities are relative newcomers to this country. These individuals present a wide range of challenges in receiving culturally competent services. The involvement of religious systems and institutions in alcohol and other drug abuse services to communities is also not without its share of challenges.

The impact of alcohol and other drug abuse on communities of color has been well documented in the popular and professional literature over the past twenty years (De La Rosa, 1998; Garcia, 1998; Gordon, 1984; Mayers, Kail and Watts, 1993; National Institute on Drug Abuse, 2003; Rebach, 1992). Communities of color have disproportionately been impacted by alcohol and other drugs. The need to have a continuum of services staffed by culturally competent staff is often mentioned as one means of meeting the needs of Latinos and other groups of color (Casas, 1992; Glick and Moore, 1990; Padilla and Snyder, 1992; Szapocznik and Kurtines, 1989). However, little attention has been paid to the potential role of religious institutions in meeting the needs of these communities within a community context that actively seeks to build upon indigenous resources (CASP, 1993). In fact, the uses of natural support systems in general, and those that are religious in particular, offer much promise for collaborative interventions with AOD organizations.

This article describes alcohol and other drug abuse and other social services provided by a religious organization (Pentecostal) in a Puerto Rican community in New England. An asset assessment was undertaken of eighteen houses of worship of which eleven agreed to be inter-viewed. Data revealed a wealth of community-based resources and the potential for collaboration between these institutions and alcohol and other drug abuse organizations. This article, as a result, sets the context for the study and provides the reader with a set of recommendations for how to involve Pentecostal organizations in collaborative activities to better reach the Puerto Rican community.

## BRIEF OVERVIEW OF LITERATURE

Any successful effort at addressing the potential role of religion in the lives of people and communities can be a tremendous task and far beyond the purposes of this article. Thus, this brief review addresses three key themes: (a) relationship between religion and alcohol and other drug abuse; (b) Puerto Rican Pentecostalism as a natural support system; and (c) barriers to collaboration between religious and human service organizations. These three areas are interrelated and will serve as a foundation from which to view an asset assessment of religious or-ganizations within a Puerto Rican community.

*Relationship Between Religion and Alcohol and Other Drug Abuse:* The professional literature on the topic of religion and substance abuse has raised important issues to be considered in how best religious orga-nizations and human service organizations can work together (CSAP, 1993). A belief in religion has been cited as a resiliency factor (North-west Regional Educational Laboratory, 1993). Hawks and Bahr (1992) found that there is a difference in frequency of alcohol use, source of al-cohol, and age of first alcohol use among various religious groups. Monteiro and Schuckit (1989) found a lower prevalence of heavy drink-ing among Jews when compared with Christian men at a university. However, Teller (1989) found that the rate of alcohol and other drug abuse is close to that of the general population, making alcohol and other drug abuse an issue among every segment of the population.

Lorch and Hughes (1988) found that fundamentalist religious groups were a significant deterrent to youth substance use/abuse. Neal's (1989) study of Black adolescents and religious involvement noted that their attendance in church significantly reduced the likelihood of alcohol use. Daily (1991) found that Seventh Day Adventist adolescents scored sig-nificantly lower on reported rates of substance use, and even lower on substance abuse, than adolescents in other Protestant churches. However, this was not the case with Latino adolescents with ethnicity being associated with higher rates of substance use.

McBridge, Mutch, Dudley and Julian's (1989) study of adult Seventh Day Adventists showed that although most adults have never used alcohol and other drugs, there is a small but growing sector of the membership that are current users. Dudley, Mutch and Cruise (1987) found that among Seventh Day Adventist youth, regular attendance in family worship was most highly associated with abstinence from alcohol and other drugs; attendance at Sabbath School first for alcohol and personal prayer first for tobacco.

The literature is quite clear about the important role religious leaders and houses of worship can play in prevention and early intervention in alcohol and other drug abuse. Brock, Key, Amuleru-Marshall, and Meehan (1990) make very strong recommendations for church involvement in all aspects of substance abuse intervention based upon the powerful role the Black church plays in the lives of countless numbers of people. Williams (1992) provides an excellent case example of how a house of worship with the proper leadership and resolve can reach communities of color. Smith (1989) stresses how human service systems have historically overlooked houses of worship as partners in prevention and treating substance abuse. Keller (1991) illustrates the role of the pastor as part of the ministry team. Scarem (1990), in turn, highlights, through personal experience, the difficulties of the recovery process and the role the church can play in helping its members in recovery.

*Puerto Rican Pentecostalism as a Natural Support System:* There is a growing body of literature analyzing the important role of religion in the lives of Puerto Ricans in the United States (Caraballo, 1990; Delgado, 1998; Delgado and Humm-Delgado, 1982; Sanchez, 1987; Sanchez-Ayendez, 1988; Stevens-Arroyo and Diaz-Stevens, 1993). The influence of Pentecostalism and other fundamentalist groups, such as Seventh Day Adventists and Jehovah's Witnesses, has been growing rapidly within this Latino group (Fitzpatrick, 1987). The popular press has captured the growing movement of Protestant denominations within the Latino community in general, and the Puerto Rican community in particular (Delgado, 1996b; Gaiter, 1980; Rohter, 1985).

Why the success of this religious movement within the Puerto Rican community? The following quotes typify why these religious organizations have made significant inroads into the Puerto Rican community: (1) "The church has become a link to their native culture–with services, then as now, conducted in Spanish–and a conduit for socialization, integration into the mainstream" (Gaiter, 1980, p. B4); (2) "Experts . . . believe that the appeal . . . is as much sociological as theological. More important than belief is belonging. . . . Newly arrived Hispanics feel uprooted and abandoned, that the rules and mores of the old world do not apply here. . . . Someone with a strong emotional charge appears and offers love, community support and an alternative to a world that no longer exists, and they move quite easily into the new matrix" (Rohter, 1985, p. 26); (3) "Many congregations offer social services such as English classes, help in finding jobs and housing, night school and drug rehabilitation programs" (Rohter, 1985, p. 26); and (4) regarding ministers–"Preachers with personal charism are everything. They earn their positions by cultivating those successful ways that attract people, hold their interest and motivate them" (Deck and Nunez, 1982, p. 232).

Caraballo (1990, p. 20), in her dissertation on this topic, raises the importance of religious organizations, in this case Pentecostal, providing a sense of community for Puerto Ricans: "The Pentecostal movement arose and survived because it serves a number of functions for the Pentecostals, for American Protestantism, and for the wider social order. The Pentecostal believer derives considerable psychic gain from religion. . . . Pentecostalism provides a catharsis for the troubled. By creating a close-knit, primary religious fellowship, it restores a sense of community to the displaced and ostracized." Consequently, Pentecostalism and other fundamentalist groups provide for expressive, informational, and instrumental needs in the Puerto Rican community and must be considered an active and influential part of any natural support system. The potential of this type of religious institution for playing a major caregiving role within the Latino community cannot be easily dismissed by the field, although achieving this goal is fraught with all kinds of challenges.

*Barriers to Collaboration Between Religious and Human Service/Alcohol and Other Drug Abuse Organizations:* The development of a constructive and mutually beneficial working relationship between these two systems (formal and natural) is a challenge (Delgado, 1994, 1996a). These two systems must overcome misperceptions, lack of trust, and very often, different worldviews and language on causation and intervention. Lenrow and Burch (1981, pp. 235-236) note a high level of distrust of professionals by religious providers which complicates development of any form of partnership: ". . . beliefs that professionals (a) are essentially exploitative, being more concerned with their economic interests and privileges than with the well-being of laypeople and the community as a whole; (b) are not competent to apply their specialized knowledge and skill to the lives of most laypeople because their understanding is limited by their academically cloistered, bureaucratically oriented, or socially privileged positions; and (c) have such limited knowledge that they frequently produce unintended and undesirable side effects . . ."

This is especially poignant in the case of social service organizations outreaching to communities of color to obtain funds without any sincere attempt to form a meaningful dialogue or collaboration. Promises may often be made before obtaining funds and totally disregarded after funds have been allocated. Instances such as these can create a tremendous amount of distrust within the community, making meaning and fruitful efforts at collaboration that much harder to achieve.

Parament (1982, p. 161), in turn, commenting on how professionals view religious-based services, states: "In recent years, professionals and social scientists have attempted to develop a greater understanding of the role social support plays in the enhancement of mental health status. Towards this end, the impact of social support systems such as the family, neighborhoods, work relationships, and self-help groups on the psychological and social well-being of people has been documented. Relatively neglected in these examinations have been the roles of religion and, more specifically, religious support systems in assisting individuals to deal with the events, problems and crises that arise in daily living."

Clearly, willingness to collaborate is no assurance of success. Consequently, any effort at development of collaborative activities must be viewed developmentally (from less to more ambitious projects), and an understanding that "testing" on both sides is to be expected and considered healthy (Delgado, 1994). This approach towards partnership helps to minimize having unrealistic expectations on both sides that can easily lead to disappointment and resentment.

## *DESCRIPTION OF SETTING AND CONTEXT OF STUDY*

The context in which religious organizations operate within becomes a critical component in better understanding why and how they go about serving their constituencies. This section, as a result, provides a foundation from which to analyze both the nature and purpose of an asset assessment of Puerto Rican Pentecostal churches. This section covers the following four areas: (a) description of site; (b) research study background and goals; (c) questionnaire construction; and (d) funding for CASP project and sub-study.

*Description of the Site:* The City of Holyoke, Massachusetts, is located approximately 100 miles west of Boston and approximately 60 miles north of Hartford, Connecticut. The city has a rich history in the textile industry, playing a prominent role in the industrial revolution. The Puerto Rican community numbers approximately 14,700 based upon the 2000 U.S. Census Bureau, and represents 36.5 percent of the total population (39,500); Puerto Ricans constituted 91.9 percent of all Latinos in the city. Holyoke is known as the Massachusetts city with the most homogeneous Latino subgroup in the state (Gaston, 1992).

The Puerto Rican community is relatively young with a median age of 18, approximately half of that of the general population. The Puerto Rican community, unfortunately, is very poor economically with a poverty rate more than four times (59.1 percent) that of white non-Latinos (13.7 percent) and African-Americans (42.8 percent); of those Puerto Ricans under the age of 18, 67.6 percent had income below the poverty level (Gaston Institute, 1994). In turning to education, Puerto Ricans lagged behind other groups in obtaining high school diplomas (60 percent had not received a high school diploma) and only 4.3 percent received a bachelor, professional or graduate degree (Gaston Institute, 1994). In essence, the Puerto Rican community in Holyoke has suffered a tremendous amount as a result of a lack of upward mobility.

*Research Study Background and Goals:* The study of Pentecostal churches was a sub-study of a broader asset assessment undertaken by ten Puerto Rican adolescents (Delgado, 1995b). This assessment gathered data on merchant/social clubs in addition to houses of worship. Unfortunately, due to a series of circumstances, e.g., hours and days of religious services, the interviewers were not able to conduct interviews of Pentecostal ministers. Lack of data on religious institutions was considered a significant shortcoming of the original study and this limitation needed to be addressed with a study specifically focused on religious institutions. As a result, an adult interviewer (supervisor of the primary asset assessment) was hired to conduct the study. This interviewer was Puerto Rican, female, and a longtime resident of Holyoke, with extensive human service experience.

A total of eighteen Pentecostal religious institutions were identified in a forty-block area of Holyoke with a large Puerto Rican representation (downtown and residential). Field interviews lasting approximately one hour were conducted with eleven ministers–seven ministers refused to participate in any aspect of the study and one only was willing to answer but just a few of the questions.

   This asset assessment of religious institutions serving the Puerto Rican community focused on three goals: (1) identify social services in general, and alcohol and other drug abuse in particular, provided by these institutions to the membership and broader community; (2) identify factors that facilitate or hinder collaboration with religious institutions; and (3) development of an asset inventory of religious institutions within a defined geographical area.

   *Questionnaire Construction:* The initial questionnaire (Religious Organization Identification) gathered data on the six generally descriptive items: (1) name of religious institution; (2) address; (3) telephone number; (4) type of church (religious affiliation); (5) size of membership; and (6) field interviewer comments/impressions. In addition to identifying information (Religious Organization Identification), the second questionnaire gathered quantitative and qualitative information on: (1) name of interviewee; (2) year church was established; (3) hours and days of operation; (4) type of social services provided; (5) leadership role in the community; and (6) comments/observations of the interviewer. Both questionnaires were in English and Spanish allowing for the interviewer to use either language, although all of the interviews were conducted in Spanish.

   *Funding for CASP Project and Sub-Study:* The Puerto Rican religious asset study was part of an overall Center on Substance Abuse Prevention project focused on high-risk Latino adolescents (Delgado, 1997). Nuevo Puente (New Bridges) was a demonstration project that linked cultural pride and substance abuse prevention. The overall goals of this CASP project were to (1) increase resiliency and protective factors to reduce the likelihood that "high-risk" youth would experiment with and become habitual users of drugs, including alcohol and tobacco; and (2) develop a community-based intervention that enriched and reinforced existing substance abuse prevention efforts by promoting acceptance of anti-substance use values and behaviors. This project was funded for a period of 3 1/2 years. The religious asset assessment, however, was funded through a non-expense extension and did not involve adolescent participants.

## FINDINGS

   Findings will be organized into three sections: (a) organizational characteristics; (b) social/alcohol and other drug abuse services, and (c) leadership role in the community. The former will provide a detailed description of eleven Pentecostal institutions and serve as a foundation from which to examine the latter. Social/alcohol and other drug abuse services, in turn, will provide data on various types and range of services provided, with particular attention to alcohol and other drug abuse. Leadership role in the community focuses on activities conducted by the ministers/churches that seek to influence the greater community in a positive manner.

*Organizational Characteristics:* The typical house of worship was Pentecostal–no Catholic or other fundamentalist churches were located within the geographical area studied, although they could be found in other sections of Holyoke. The typical Pentecostal church had been in existence for six years. However, this average of six years is based on ten churches; one church (Salvation Army affiliated) had been in existence for 100 years and was not founded by the Puerto Rican community and was not included in the average because of the unique set of circumstances surrounding its origin.

Churches were in operation from a period of less than one year (N = 2) to 20 years or more (N = 1). However, most of the churches (N = 7) were fairly new to the city with less than four years of existence. This increase in popularity parallels what has been reported in the popular press–namely, Pentecostals have made significant progress in attracting Puerto Ricans/Latinos to their religious movement.

Membership size also differed considerably and ranged from 25 to 200 members; the latter church also had the longest longevity of all the churches (established in 1970). The average membership was 71; most of the churches, however, had 75 or less members. Caraballo's (1990) study of twenty-eight Boston-based Pentecostal churches noted a membership range of 27 to 93 and an average size of 56. The Holyoke sample, as a result, represents a significantly larger membership even though the Puerto Rican/Latino community is much smaller numerically than that of Boston with approximately 62,000 of which 25,700 were Puerto Rican. Interestingly, there were no major patterns associated with longevity. One of the churches with the shortest longevity (established in 1993) had seventy members and one of the longest (1982) had the same number of members.

In turning to hours of operation, the average was ten hours per week and it ranged from 1 1/4 (membership of 50 and established in 1992) to 15 hours (membership of 120 and established in 1979). Most of the churches were opened six to ten hours (N = 4) and eleven to fifteen hours (N = 6). Consequently, the Pentecostal churches in the Holyoke sample had very limited number of hours of operation, with the majority devoted to religious masses.

Only one church was open seven days per week and one was open just one day per week; the average number of days open was approximately four days per week ($\times$ 4.3 days). Sundays were the most frequently open day with all churches providing services; this day was followed by Thursday (N = 10) and Friday (N = 10). Tuesday (N = 7), Monday (N = 5), Wednesday (N = 3) and Saturday (N = 1) followed in popularity. The combination of Monday, Thursday, Friday and Sunday were the most frequently cited combination of days (N = 5). Caraballo's study (1990) reflected similar findings with the average Pentecostal institution in Boston being opened four days. However, the most popular combination of days differed slightly from that of Holyoke–Tuesday, Thursday, Friday and Sunday.

A multidimensional perspective is needed to better understand the Pentecostal churches in the sample. The two churches with the longest longevity (15 and 24 years respectively) and the largest membership (120 and 200 members) were also opened the longest period of time (15 and 14 hours). However, the church with the smallest membership (25 members) and the relatively shortest period of existence (1 1/2 years) was not too far behind these two institutions, with a total of 12 hours of operation. Generally speaking, institutions with the largest membership have also been in existence the longest period of time, had the highest number of operating hours, and were open the most days.

*Social/Alcohol and Other Drug Abuse Services:* As highlighted in the professional literature, Pentecostal churches serve a vital function in meeting the spiritual, social, psychological, and physical needs of its membership. One of the goals of this study was to identify the social/alcohol and other drug abuse services provided by churches. A total of sixteen social services were identified addressing informational, instrumental, and expressive needs of the members. The average Pentecostal church provided approximately seven social/alcohol and other drug abuse services ($\times$ 7.3) and ranged from a low of three (N = 1) to a high of eleven services (N = 1). Interestingly, the largest and second largest churches in terms of membership did not offer the most services. The Pentecostal church offering the most services (N = 10) had a membership of 80 and was opened 9 1/2 hours and four days per week. However, it had the longest longevity of the ten churches established by Puerto Ricans (20 years). The two newest churches with three and four types provided the fewest number of services respectively.

Friendship for the lonely (social activities and a drop-in service) was the service provided by almost all of the churches (N = 10). This service was followed in popularity by provision of food for the hungry (donations and meals) and interpreter services (both were listed nine times). The latter service entailed a minister or other church members going with individuals to agencies, etc., to aid them in seeking services by serving as interpreters for those with minimal or no English language skills.

Eight Pentecostal churches listed financial assistance and counseling. The former entailed loans, donations, to help members in financial crisis and the latter was a service provided for membership with familial/alcohol and other drug abuse problems; it should be noted that individual/families with severe emotional problems might be referred to human service organizations. This finding corroborates that of the Caraballo study (1990)–namely, ministers (21 out of 28) reported making referrals to appropriate mental health/social service agencies if the presenting problem was too great. Surprisingly, provision of transportation (attending services and appointments) was only listed by two institutions; the Caraballo (1990) study found that all twenty-eight churches provided this service (vehicle provided by the church itself or the membership). Home visiting for the frail/sick and English classes were only cited once each in the Holyoke study.

In turning to alcohol and other drug abuse specific services, only five institutions indicated that they had or currently have services for individuals in recovery and their families. One institution noted that it had a large number of members with human service/alcohol and other drug abuse backgrounds and this facilitated the meeting of membership alcohol and other drug abuse needs. Another institution indicated that it had a residential program for individuals in recovery. One institution used to provide alcohol and other drug abuse services prior to moving to a new location–lack of space did not permit offering this type of service.

Finally, two institutions noted that they provided some or all of the following: support groups for family members, counseling for individuals in recovery, skill development workshops (i.e., self-esteem development, refusal skills). The Caraballo study (1990) had similar findings. Only seven out of the twenty-eight Pentecostal churches provided alcohol and other drug abuse-related services; most of the ministers (21 out of 28) could not identify an alcohol and other drug abuse treatment facility in order to make a referral.

*Leadership Role in the Community:* Ministers were asked about the leadership role of the church in the greater community. Only two out of the ten ministers who answered this question indicated they did not play leadership roles in the community. These two churches were only recently established (1 1/2 years and 2 months) and did not have the resources/capacity/time to play influential roles within the community; the remaining eight churches indicated some form of leadership role. Roles varied, however, and generally entailed any one or combination of the following: (1) provision of workshop leaders/speakers on various topics; (2) sponsoring sporting/recreational activities; (3) participation in peace/anti-racism rallies/marches; (4) radio programming on topics of community interests; (5) operation of food pantries; (6) community-oriented conferences on family/youth themes; (7) participation on community agency boards or advisory committees; (8) sponsoring and participating in community clean-up/safe street activities; and (9) folkloric dancers/band for community festivals.

The above listing reflects a wide range of community-leadership activities. The larger and more established churches played a more prominent leadership role based upon the number of activities listed; as already noted, the newer churches did not due to start-up organizational demands. Leadership roles offer tremendous potential for churches to both recruit new members and influence community-wide issues.

## RECOMMENDATIONS

The role of twelve-step programs in the field of alcohol and other drug abuse has been well established (Katz, 1993). The movement towards cultural competence in the field of alcohol and other drug abuse/human services (Cross, 1988; Gordon, 1994) has highlighted the importance of religion and religious beliefs as a vital part of any effort to bring multicultural concepts into practice (Pate and Bondi, 1992; Pederson, 1991; Stander, Piercy, Mackinnon and Helmeke, 1994). The following recommendations cover a wide range of activities, with varying degrees of difficult and labor intensity. Recommendations fall into seven categories (Lee, 1994): (1) training; (2) provision of alcohol and other drug abuse information; (3) resource utilization; (4) promoting alternatives through community education; (5) enhancing social competence; (6) policy development; and (7) guiding principles.

*Training:* The provision of training represents one method of maximizing limited resources. There is no question that ministers are important community impactors; consequently, it is necessary to assess their needs in the field of alcohol and other drug abuse and provide necessary support through training and consultation. Increasing their competence to assess alcohol and other drug abuse needs and, if necessary, make referrals to appropriate agencies, will represent an important step in the development of collaboration between churches and agencies. However, it would be a tremendous mistake to conceptualize training as strictly one-sided–namely, professionals helping those who are "less" professional. As a result, ministers and key church members can also serve to train alcohol and other drug abuse/agency staff in the methods they use to reach and help the membership. Training is generally not labor intensive and can serve as an excellent foundation for more ambitious collaborative projects once there is a relationship built on trust.

*Provision of Alcohol and Other Drug Abuse Information:* The results of the asset assessment uncovered a need for alcohol and other drug abuse information in Spanish. Most of the ministers were not addressing alcohol and other drug abuse issues within their membership and in the general community. This, as already indicated, is similar to the Caraballo (1990) findings. Consequently, the development and distribution of alcohol and other drug abuse material can represent a crucial initial step in highlighting the alcohol and other drug abuse needs of the membership. Information can also be distributed in video as long as it is in Spanish with English subtitles.

An advisory committee composed of ministers and other key religious leaders can provide alcohol and other drug abuse agencies with valuable input into the development of material (print and visual) that specifically targets memberships. Church officials, in turn, if available, share with agencies materials they have developed and how and when they are used with the membership. It is important to always keep in mind the spirit of collaboration–two sides share and benefit.

*Resource Utilization:* The utilization of religious personnel/counselors as allies, if appropriate, is not that unusual in the field of human services (Pate and Bondi, 1992). This can be particularly advantageous in situations where a church member may be utilizing a variety of social services. Consequently, it is necessary for alcohol and other drug abuse and other human service agencies to gather information on client belief systems and religious practices; this information can serve as a foundation for development of collaborative services. Churches must be a part of any resource directory on community resources, for example. This takes on added importance when there is a lack of bilingual and bicultural staff/resources; in short, human service organizations do not have the luxury of limiting their view of what is a "proper" resource.

In turning to use of physical resources, there is an excellent potential for alcohol and other drug abuse agencies to utilize church space for conducting training groups, meetings, etc. These churches, invariably, are located within the community and are geographically accessible. Agencies, in turn, can make space available for large community meetings, training sessions, etc. Agencies can develop referral processes with churches for those instances where a member's needs are beyond the competence of church officials. This process can be simplified and involve a contact person in the organization who is well known, respected, and versed on religious practices.

Agencies can take advantage of an invaluable human resource that ministers represent. Organizations can hire ministers into professional positions such as co-leaders of groups, intake workers, overnight staff and therapists (when qualified); ministers can undertake internships to help them learn interviewing and counseling skills that can be of benefit to clients, congregations, and the community in general. Ministers can serve as effective advocates for a community, particularly when they are part of a coalition with providers.

*Promoting Alternatives Through Community Education:* The undertaking of community education involving co-sponsorship offers a richness of possibilities for establishing and maintaining collaborative partnerships with houses of worship such as those in this study. Several of the churches in the study undertook community conferences or had radio programs; consequently, this offers an excellent opportunity for collaboration or the provision of "expert" speakers on a variety of alcohol and other drug abuse topics.

Community conferences, in turn, provide a tremendous amount of visibility for all collaborating parties and can serve a unifying role within the community. In addition, these activities are not necessarily labor intensive and can serve as vehicles for identifying other community needs. There are relatively few venues within a community for the entire community, including providers, to come together to share and engage in dialogue. Conferences, when well planned and implemented, are such forums.

*Enhancing Social Competence:* Several ministers indicated that they offered workshops that enhanced social competence among the membership; some of these workshops focused specifically on youth. The provision of workshop leaders (co-leaders) represents a cost-effective manner of reaching a large population. Alcohol and other drug abuse agencies can also offer these workshops in their settings and invite members from a variety of churches to participate. Much has been learned in the field about skill development (Van Hasselt, De Piano and Tarter, 1994), and this knowledge can be shared with ministers and other church personnel. Alcohol and other drug abuse staff, in turn, will derive considerable benefits from the knowledge they obtain as a result of leading, or co-leading, these workshops.

*Policy Development:* There is little doubt that ministers and other church officials must be included in any coalition/task forces focused on helping the community. However, we must also seek to involve them on agency boards of directors, advisory committees, etc., because they represent an important perspective on community needs. Churches, in turn, may wish to establish advisory committees composed of members and outside participants to help them establish or maintain alcohol and other drug abuse and other services. Input from both of these parties will increase the likelihood that policy development reflects the culture-specific needs of the community.

*Guiding Principles:* In working with ministers, it is important to be mindful of a number of guiding principles designed to enhance the collaborative process. These principles include: (1) Develop a sense of trust among the collaborating entities that is based on mutual respect; (2) Develop a clear understanding of the concerns of congregations and demonstrate a willingness to address those issues; (3) Avoid paternalism by forming a relationship of co-learners in which both the perspective and knowledge of all collaborators are acknowledged; (4) Understand that forming a partnership can be a complex process in which both parties must continually re-examine and re-evaluate the nature of the relationship; (5) Limit the bureaucratic demands placed on ministers since most have limited administrative support staff (or none at all); and (6) Accept that turf issues are inherent in collaborations, yet find ways to develop ways to work together for the common good.

## *CONCLUSION*

This article has provided the reader with a brief glimpse into an important religious support system within the Puerto Rican community. However, the implications of this support system goes far beyond the impact on one ethnic group; this support system touches the lives of countless numbers in the United States. Resources that specifically target alcohol and other drug abuse needs in communities of color are not sufficient to meet the needs of these communities. In addition, the provision of services within a cultural context necessitates the development of "innovative" strategies that are not only community-based but also serve to tap indigenous community resources whenever possible and applicable.

The involvement of Pentecostal churches in collaborative activities with alcohol and other drug abuse/human service organizations has its challenges, as evidenced by the high refusal rate in this study (7 out of 18). However, this reluctance to get involved must not dissuade organizations from seeking collaborative ventures with churches. It does raise, however, the importance of viewing collaboration within a developmental framework that builds upon previous work together and the goodwill and reputations that emerge as a result.

The alcohol and other drug abuse field must endeavor to explore new ways of involving undervalued communities; utilization of natural resources and community capacity development offers much promise for the field and communities of color. The information presented in this article represents an initial step in the direction of bringing together two worlds (natural and formal) in an effort to have communities better address the needs of their members.

## REFERENCES

Caraballo, E.R. (1990). *The role of the Pentecostal church as a service provider in the Puerto Rican community in Boston, Massachusetts: A case study.* Waltham, MA: Doctoral Dissertation, Brandeis University.

Casas, J.M. (1992). A culturally sensitive model for evaluating alcohol and other drug abuse prevention programs: A Hispanic perspective. In M.A. Orlandi, R. Weston, and L.G. Epstein (Eds.), *Cultural competence for evaluators* (pp. 75-116). Rockville, MD: Office of Substance Abuse Prevention.

Center on Substance Abuse Prevention. (1993). *Faith Communities.* Rockville, MD: U.S. Department of Health and Human Services.

Cross, T.L (1988). Services to minority populations. *Focal Point,* 3, 1-4.

Daily, S.G. (1991). *Adventist adolescents and addiction: Substance use/abuse in an adventist population and its relationship to religion, family, self-perception, and deviant behavior.* Dissertation Abstracts International, 52B, 3315B-3316B.

Deck, A.F. and Nunez, J.A. (1982). Religious enthusiasm and Hispanic youth. *America,* October 23, 232-234.

De La Rosa, M. (1998). Prevalence and consequences of alcohol, cigarette, and drug use among Hispanics. *Alcoholism Treatment Quarterly,* 16, 21-54.

De La Rosa, M., Segal, B., and Lopez, R. (Eds.). *Conducting drug abuse research with minority populations: Advances and issues.* New York: Haworth Press.

Delgado, M. (1998). Religion as a caregiving system for Puerto Rican elders with functional disabilities. In M. Delgado (Ed.), *Social services in Latino communities: Research and strategies* (pp. 35-50). New York: Haworth Press.

Delgado, M. (1997). Strengths-based practice with Puerto Rican adolescents: Lessons from a substance abuse prevention project. *Social Work in Education*, 19, 101-112.

Delgado, M. (1996a). Implementing a natural support system AOD project: Administrative considerations and recommendations. *Alcoholism Treatment Quarterly*, 14, 1-14.

Delgado, M. (1996b). Puerto Rican natural support systems and the field of AOD: Implications for religious institutions. *Journal of Ministry in Addiction & Recovery*, 3, 67-77.

Delgado, M. (1995a). Hispanic natural support systems and the AOD field: Issues and challenges. *Alcoholism Treatment Quarterly*, 12, 17-32.

Delgado, M. (1995b). Community asset assessment and substance abuse prevention: A case study involving the Puerto Rican community. *Journal of Child and Adolescent Substance Abuse*, 4, 57-77.

Delgado, M. (1994). Collaboration between Hispanic natural support systems and AOD agencies: A developmental perspective. *Journal of Multicultural Social Work*, 3, 11-37.

Delgado, M. and Humm-Delgado, D. (1981). Natural support systems: Source of strength in Hispanic communities. *Social Work*, 1982, 27, 83-89.

Duley, R.L., Mutch, P.B., and Cruise, R.J. (1987). Religious factors and drug usage among Seventh-Day Adventist youth in North America. *Journal for the Scientific Study of Religion*, 26, 218-223.

Fitzpatrick, J.P. (1987). *Puerto Rican Americans: The meaning of migration to the mainland.* Englewood Cliffs, NJ: Prentice-Hall Publishers.

Gaiter, D.J. (December 24, 1980). At Christmas, Hispanic Pentecostal church puts stress on 'gifts' without price tags. *The New York Times*, B1, B4.

Garcia, B. (1998). Professional development of AODA practice with Latinos: The utility of supervision, in-service training and consultation. *Alcoholism Treatment Quarterly*, 16, 85-108.

Gaston Institute. (1992). *Latinos in Holyoke.* Boston, MA: University of Massachusetts.

Gaston Institute. (1994). *Latinos in Holyoke: Poverty, income, education, employment, and housing.* Boston, MA: University of Massachusetts.

Glick, R. and Moore, J. (Eds.) (1980). *Drugs in Hispanic communities.* New Brunswick, NJ: Rutgers University Press.

Gordon, J.U. (Ed.) (1994). *Managing multiculturalism in substance abuse services.* Thousand Oaks, CA: Sage Publications.

Hawks, R.D. and Bahr, S.H. (1992). Religion and drug use. *Journal of Drug Education*, 22, 1-8.

Keller, J.E. (1991). *Alcoholics & their families: Guide for clergy & congregations.* New York: Harper Collins Publishers.

Lee, J.M. (1994). Historical and theoretical considerations: Implications for multiculturalism in substance abuse services. In J.U. Gordon (Ed.), *Managing multiculturalism in substance abuse services* (pp. 3-21). Thousand Oaks, CA: Sage Publications.

Lenrow, P.B. and Burch, R.W. (1981). Mutual aid and professional services: Opposing or complimentary, In B.H. Gottlieb (Ed.), *Social networks and social support* (pp. 233-257). Beverly Hills, CA: Sage Publications.

Lorch, B.R. and Hughes, R.H. (1988). Church, youth, alcohol, and educational programs and youth substance use. *Journal of Alcohol and Drug Education*, 33, 14-26.

Mayers, R.S., Kail, B.L., and Watts, T.D. (Eds.). (1993). *Hispanic substance abuse.* Springfield, IL: Charles C. Thomas Press.

McBride, D.C., Mutch, P.B., Dudley, R.L., and Julian, A.G. (1989). Substance use and correlates among adult Seventh-Day Adventists in North America. As reported in *Faith communities* (p. 17). Rockville, MD: U.S. Development of Health and Human Services.

Monteiro, M.G. and Schuckitt, M.A. (1989). Alcohol, drug and mental health problems among Jewish and Christian men at a university. *American Journal of Drug and Alcohol Abuse,* 15, 403-412.

National Institute on Drug Abuse. (2003). *Drug use among racial/ethnic minorities.* Rockville, MD: Author.

Neal, A.A. (1989). *Religious involvement and practices concerning the use of alcohol among black adolescents.* Dissertation Abstracts International, 49, 4256-B-4257-B.

Northwest Regional Educational Laboratory. (1993). *Using community-wide collaboration to foster resiliency in kids: A conceptual framework.* Portland, Oregon.

Padilla, A.M. and Synder, V.N.S. (1992). Hispanics: What the culturally informed evaluator needs to know. In M.A. Orlandi, R. Weston, and L. G. Epstein (Eds.), *Cultural competence for evaluators* (pp. 117-146). Rockville, MD: Office of Substance Abuse Prevention.

Pargament, K.I. (1982). The interface among religion, religious support systems, and mental health. In D.E. Biegel and A.J. Naparstek (Eds.), *Community support systems and mental health* (pp. 161-174). New York: Springer Publishing Co.

Pate, Jr., R.H. and Bondi, A.M. (1992). Religious beliefs and practice: An integral aspect of multi-cultural awareness. *Counselor Education and Supervision,* 32, 108-115.

Pedersen, P. (Ed.), (1991). Multiculturalism as a fourth force in counseling (Special Issue). *Journal of Counseling and Development,* 70, entire issue.

Rashid, H., Brock, R., Key, A., Amuleru-Marshall, and Meehan, S. (1990). Prevention models for black youth at high risk: Family and religion. In U.J. Oyemade and D. Brandon-Monye (Eds.), *Ecology of alcohol and other drug use: Helping Black high risk youth* (pp. 134-150). Rockville, MD: Office for Substance Abuse Prevention.

Rebach, H. (1992). Alcohol and drug use among American minorities. In J.E. Trimble, C.S. Bolek, and S.J. Niemcryk (Eds.), *Ethnic and multi-cultural drug abuse* (pp. 23-57). Binghamton, NY: Harrington Park Press.

Rohter, L. (Saturday, January 12, 1985). Protestantism gaining influence in Hispanic community. *The New York Times,* pp. 23, 26.

Sanchez, C. (1987). Self-help: Model for strengthening the informal support system of the Hispanic elderly. *Journal of Gerontological Social Work,* 9, 117-130.

Sanchez Ayendez, M. (1988). Puerto Rican elderly women: The cultural dimension of social support network. *Women & Health,* 14, 239-252.

Scarem, R.H., Jr. (1989). *Minister equipped for facilitating alcoholism recovery in and through a Christian church: A journey.* Dissertation Abstracts International, 49, 2693-A.

Smith, D. (1989). An overlooked resource. *Alcoholism and Addiction,* November, pp. 4-8.

Stander, V., Piercy, F.P., Mackinnon, D., and Helmeke, K. (1994). Spirituality, religion, and family therapy: Competing or complementary worlds. *The American Journal of Family Therapy,* 22, 27-40.

Stevens-Arroyo, A.M. and Diaz-Stevens, A.M. (1993). Latino churches and schools as urban battlefields. In S.W. Rothstein (Ed.), *Handbook of schooling in urban America.* Westport, CT: Greenwood Press.

Szapocnik, J. and Kurtines, W.M. (Eds.). (1989). *Breakthroughs in family therapy with drug-abusing and problem youth.* New York: Springer Publishing Co.

Teller, B. (1989). Chemical dependency in the Jewish community. *The Counselor,* May/June, pp. 17-20.

Van Hasselt, V.B., De Piano, F. and Tarter, R.E. (1994). Overview and statement of purpose. *Journal of Child & Adolescent Substance Abuse,* 3, 1-11.

Williams, C. (1992). *No hiding place: Empowerment and recovery for our troubled communities.* New York: Harper Collins Publishers.

# SECTION 3:
# SUMMARY OF PREVENTION
# AND TREATMENT IMPLICATIONS

## Chapter 12

# Cross-Cutting Themes
# and Recommendations

Melvin Delgado, PhD

**SUMMARY.** The authors in this volume have done an outstanding job raising awareness of the challenges that lay before us in better serving Latinos in the field of alcohol and providing action steps to help us achieve the goals associated with culturally competent practice. There is little doubt that the next decade will bring with it a host of opportunities and challenges as Latinos continue their dramatic numerical increase throughout all regions of this country. *[Article copies available for a fee from The Haworth Document Delivery Service: 1-800-HAWORTH. E-mail address: <docdelivery@haworthpress.com> Website: <http://www.HaworthPress.com> © 2005 by The Haworth Press, Inc. All rights reserved.]*

Melvin Delgado is Professor of Social Work and Chair of Macro-Practice at Boston University School of Social Work, 264 Bay State Road, Boston, MA 02215.

[Haworth co-indexing entry note]: "Cross-Cutting Themes and Recommendations." Delgado, Melvin. Co-published simultaneously in *Alcoholism Treatment Quarterly* (The Haworth Press, Inc.) Vol. 23, No. 2/3, 2005, pp. 205-212; and: *Latinos and Alcohol Use/Abuse Revisited: Advances and Challenges for Prevention and Treatment Programs* (ed: Melvin Delgado) The Haworth Press, Inc., 2005, pp. 205-212. Single or multiple copies of this article are available for a fee from The Haworth Document Delivery Service [1-800-HAWORTH, 9:00 a.m. - 5:00 p.m. (EST). E-mail address: docdelivery@haworthpress.com].

Available online at http://www.haworthpress.com/web/ATQ
© 2005 by The Haworth Press, Inc. All rights reserved.
doi:10.1300/J020v23n02_12

**KEYWORDS.** Latinos, prevention, treatment

The field of alcohol services and research will face considerable challenges in the next two decades as evidenced by what has been encountered over the past two decades (McGovern & White, 2002). One set of challenges is how to put the social problems associated with alcohol in the public domain so that funding of services, research, and scholarship can operate fairly alongside other drugs such as heroin and cocaine. However, just as important is how do we in the field manage the resources we do have to better reach many underrepresented groups such as Latinos and the numerous and ever expanding subgroups of this population? These two critical challenges, however, are not mutually exclusive yet speak well to what the field needs to accomplish in the next decade.

This volume as noted in the introductory article has sought to move the field further along in search of models for accessing the Latino community in this country. In so doing, serious questions and issues have been raised directly and indirectly with how the problems associated with Latinos and alcohol are conceptualized and addressed in the field. The question of how best to address the alcohol and other drug abuse needs of Latinos needs to be couched within a broader set of questions and themes to better contextualize the factors precipitating use of alcohol and other drugs and how best to address them.

The following seven themes/questions have been developed as a creative way of identifying the key issues and recommendations that cut across the articles in this volume. Each of these themes/questions attempts to identify key challenges and proposes strategies to help the field move closer towards achieving culturally competent services within the Latino community. A word of caution is in order, however. The editor takes full responsibility for identifying and framing these themes/questions and the writers of the articles may, or may not, agree with these selections. The reader, too, may well argue for the substituting of themes they believe is the most pressing. Such a perspective is not only welcomed but also encouraged and bodes well for moving the field forward in a progressive manner.

The field of alcohol services cannot afford the "luxury" of ignoring current demographic trends and how best to position itself in the immediate. Disregarding or minimizing the needs of Latinos can prove disastrous when the field finally decides that it is time to move in a progressive manner to meet the needs of this ever-expanding community.

Treatment failures are well recognized by the community and creation of a state of mind of distrust of the field can seriously hamper Latinos in need seeking services.

1. *"If we build the program, will they come?"* The age-old question of which comes first–the chicken or the egg applies to culture-competent programming. In programming and services terms, does demand bring about services or must services first be in place to create demand? Thus, the question of how to increase meaningful outreach and engagement, or access if you wish, of Latinos runs throughout all of the articles in this volume. Each of these articles is quick, however, to acknowledge the challenges that lay before us in better serving Latinos. Culturally competent delivery of alcohol and other drug abuse services is predicated on a number of key principles pertaining to access.

Access, however, is a complex construct that at minimum must take into account four distinct yet interrelated aspects. Each of these aspects is of equal importance: (1) geographic; (2) psychological; (3) cultural; and (4) operational. Geographic access refers to the distance a consumer must travel and the difficulty of negotiating public transportation to receive services. Very often geographic accessibility is substituted with availability of services. Although geographic accessibility is very important, it would be too simplistic to equate these two concepts without considering other dimensions.

Psychological accessibility refers to the stigma that is associated with service utilization. Thus, a service may be accessible geographically as in the case where an outpost or satellite office is placed within the Latino community but it is so stigmatizing to go there that for all intents and purposes it could be located a thousand miles away. Few individuals will be willing to risk their reputations seeking services there. Cultural accessibility refers to an organization's ability to provide services in the preferred language of the consumer and systematically incorporates key cultural values and beliefs into the services being provided. Finally, logistical accessibility refers to the hours and days of operation. Life in a community is never conceptualized and lived on a 9 a.m. to 5 p.m. schedule, five days per week (Monday through Friday). Thus, programs must endeavor to broaden the operational period to include evenings, weekends and holidays.

The diversity of the Latino community is not new. However, its extent is unparalleled in this nation's history. Thus, service accessibility as a result must reach beyond traditional boundaries and incorporate innovative and cultural perspectives throughout all facets of programming. Failure to do so ultimately means that the Latino community cannot possibly access themselves of valuable resources to treat a major social problem. Any effective model that is developed for reaching Latinos will almost certainly be dated by the time it appears in scholarly print. That is to be expected and must be the goal, challenging and frustrating as that may be!

2. *"The more we change, the more we need to change."* The tremendous demographic changes specifically addressed by Ms. Miranda but also evident in many of the other articles necessitate the alcohol-related services be ever willing to change to take into account many of the issues associated with provision of culturally competent services. The days of just listing on an intake form, for example, that the consumer was Latino/a, will no longer be sufficient (Rodriguez-Andrew, 1998).

It is also necessary to venture out of the conventional categories and take into account the migration journey and the circumstances surrounding their stay in this country. A Latino who is born and raised in this country will have a different world experience from one who is an immigrant with requisite immigration papers. Their experience would be dramatically different to that of a Latino who is in this country without legal documentation. Thus, it means that we must be prepared to broaden the kind of information that we gather through intake and intervention and take into consideration a host of social-political factors in the process of doing so. This information, in turn, must influence how we conceptualize and deliver services.

The expectation that programming and services are to be dynamic and willing to change to accommodate new groups should not be a principle that can be labeled as "radical." Communities are dynamic in character and so should the programs that serve them. Nevertheless, when this principle is translated into services for the Latino community it means that staff must reflect the population we are serving, in-service training to increase the knowledge base and competencies of staff to address new challenges (Garcia, 1998).

3. *"The community is out there, and what do we do with it?"* The continued recommendation of structuring services in such a way as to involve the community is not new. However, the presence of natural support systems and other cultural resources firmly based outside of conventional alcohol-related programs, requires that we find creative ways of bringing these resources into the prevention and treatment arenas (Delgado, 1998). Success in doing so will be measured by the amount of time, energy, and resources that will be marshaled into this goal. However, there really is no shortcut in accomplishing community involvement (Delgado, 1999a,b).

Further, although it is quite fashionable to romanticize community and I have certainly been accused, and rightly, of doing so, there are many consequences associated with community involvement. Latino communities are never homogeneous. Some groups have long histories of distrust and conflicts with other groups prior to arrival in this country. These tensions and negative perceptions were not left at the borders of this country upon their entry and we can find them still prevalent in the community.

Bridging the gap between community and community-based treatment will facilitate the undertaking of research, qualitative as well as quantitative, to better assist us in understanding the role of alcohol in the life of the Latino community (De La Rosa, Segal & Lopez, 1999; Institute of Medicine, 1998). Increasing the knowledge base on the subject of alcohol and Latinos necessitates a close and trusting relationship between the Latino community, its community-based organizations, and academia. Achieving these types of partnerships, however, will not be easy (Massey, Ortiz & Alex, 1999).

4. *"Alcohol and what else?"* The subject of alcohol use and abuse can no longer be viewed in isolation from the use of other drugs, including tobacco. Neither should this subject be viewed narrowly by focusing on one type of alcohol beverage. The interplay between alcohol and other drugs effectively means that any prevention campaign focusing on mass media, for example, is doomed to fail if it misses the target–namely, there is simply not one drug being abused. There certainly may be a primary drug of preference. However, it does not mean that other drugs are not part of the landscape.

The findings from Dr. Lundgren and colleagues' study raise important questions for the field of alcohol and have implications for service delivery focused on Latinos. Although the Massachusetts study cannot be generalized beyond a certain population group of Latinos, in this case Puerto Rican, it nonetheless raises important questions for us pertaining to the role of alcohol in the life of heroin users.

5. *"Where do prisons and jails fall within a comprehensive system of care?"* The disturbing but nevertheless real trend towards incarceration in this country has direct implications for the field of alcohol and other drug abuse treatment. Dr. Garcia has put forth a powerful agenda for better serving the needs of Latinas within the correctional system. Latinos, too, are in desperate need for services while incarcerated and after reentry back into the community.

Alcohol and other drug abuse if left untreated, as is often the case in a criminal justice system where demand for these types of services far outstrip available resources, does not bode well. Any effort for Latinas to be reunited with their children and families can best be considered the unrealization of their dream. Not because this is not a primary goal in their lives, but because treatment has not been readily available during a time period when they are most amendable to receiving it.

The relative youthfulness of the Latino community in this country can be both an asset as well as a liability. Youth have a higher likelihood of engaging in risk-taking behaviors that can land them in the correctional system. Once in this system they are also more likely to have a high rate of recidivism and engage in excessive drinking and other drug use, not to mention that from a health standpoint these institutions are toxic (Delgado & Humm-Delgado, in press). This necessitates that active efforts at prevention and early intervention take on greater prominence with Latinos than with other groups of color in the United States. The criminal justice system, as noted by Dr. Pabon, covers a wide stretch of ages with Latino youth playing an increasingly larger role in service utilization within these systems.

Latino/a involvement in gangs brings with it a host of challenges for prevention and treatment of alcohol-related problems and issues. The possibility of actively reaching out to gang members is not without its share of concerns for the safety of staff and fears of alienating other consumers of services who fear association with a program that has former or current gang members. Nevertheless, the field of alcohol and other drug abuses can ill-afford to turn its back on this population group which tends to be relatively young. If so, it will only be a question of time before these individuals, males and females, find their way into the criminal justice system with all of its deleterious consequences for the Latino community.

6. *"Where are Latino natural support systems in this equation?"* One persistent theme throughout all of the articles has been the importance of cultural resources in the planning and delivery of alcohol-related services (Delgado & Humm-Delgado, 1993; Rodriguez-Andrew, 1998). As already noted in Question 1, engagement of Latinos will require that organizations actively seek to build their programs tapping community cultural resources (Brandes, 2002). These resources can be viewed from a variety of perspectives–instrumental (concrete ways that they can assist), expressive (emotional/political support), and informational (the latest perspective on issues and how best to engage various sectors of the community).

Family is without question at the center of any form of natural support system although challenges uplifted in this volume raise critical questions about the ultimate outcome of Latino families in this society. Dr. Vega and colleague and Dr. Bullock, for example, provide important but disturbing consequences of how life in this society gets even more complicated for Latinos when alcohol and other drug abuse are part of their life.

The construct of a natural support system was evident in the articles and the importance in any effort to contextualize the findings of the research and develop any form of culturally competent initiatives. This is not to say that Latino communities can simply address their own needs with their own resources. That would be blaming the victim and further victimizing them when they cannot succeed. However, it does lead to the need to develop initiatives that systematically incorporate natural support systems whenever possible.

7. *"Researchers, who needs them?"* This volume cannot but help raise the importance of research in better informing the field of practice. Unfortunately, researchers have developed a very negative reputation in many quarters, and to be quite honest, well deserved. However, the authors of the articles in this volume symbolize the important work that can transpire when researchers take a culturally competent perspective towards this activity (Cervantes & Pena, 1998).

It is unreasonable to expect practitioners to take time from their busy schedules to pause, reflect, and initiate investigations. Those tasks are within the scope of an active research agenda. However, it would be unreasonable for researchers to simply view their activities aside of the needs and agendas of practitioners. In short, a partnership needs to be developed that is based upon mutual trust and respect. This, I am afraid, will take time and considerable effort but I see this collaboration as the only way that the field can truly respond to the current and emerging needs of Latinos and other marginalized groups in this society.

## *CONCLUSION*

It is arduous to imagine that this is the conclusion to the final chapter of this volume. This volume required several years of planning and carrying out numerous tasks. Special issues like edited books necessitate that editors possess a vision of what they wish the final "product" to be and have the patience, and connections, to carry out this vision. This volume truly reflects this point.

The reader can no doubt surmise the enjoyment I had in writing this final chapter. This sense of "fun" is not because the volume is complete but because the authors of the articles did such a thoughtful and competent job of writing them. This made writing this chapter relatively easy to accomplish but also raised for me the distance we still need to travel to make the field of alcohol services accessible to the rapidly changing Latino community in the early part of the twenty-first century!

## REFERENCES

Brandes, S. (2002). *Staying sober in Mexico City*. Austin, TX: University of Texas Press.

Cervantes, R.C. & Pena, C. (1998). Evaluating Hispanic/Latino programs: Ensuring cultural competence. *Alcoholism Treatment Quarterly*, 16, pp.109-131.

De La Rosa, M., Segal, B. & Lopez, R. (Eds.). *Conducting drug abuse research with minority populations: Advances and issues*. New York: Haworth Press.

Delgado, M. (1999a). Involvement of the Hispanic community in ATOD research. In M. De La Rosa, B. Segal, & R. Lopez. (Eds.). *Conducting drug abuse research with minority populations: Advances and issues* (pp.93-105). New York: Haworth Press.

Delgado, M. (1999b). A state of the art review of Latinos and substance abuse. In S.B. Kar (Ed.). *Substance abuse prevention: A multicultural perspective* (pp.155-170). Amityville, NY: Baywood Publishing Co., Inc.

Delgado, M. (1998). Alcoholism services and community settings: Latina beauty parlors as case examples. *Alcoholism Treatment Quarterly*, 16, pp.71-83.

Delgado, M. & Humm-Delgado, D. (In Press). *Health and health care in the nation's prisons: Issues, challenges, and policies*. Westport, CT: Praeger Publishers.

Delgado, M. & Humm-Delgado, D. (1993). Chemical dependence, self-help groups, and the Hispanic community. In R. Sanchez-Mayers, B. Kail & T. Watts (Eds.). *Hispanic substance abuse* (pp.145-156). Springfield, IL: Charles C. Thomas.

Garcia, B. (1998). Professional development of AODA practice with Latinos: The utility of supervision, in-service training and consultation. *Alcoholism Treatment Quarterly*, 16, pp.85-108.

Institute of Medicine. (1998). *Bridging the gap between practice and research: Forging partnerships with community-based drug and alcohol treatment*. Washington, D.C.: National Academy Press.

Massey, E., Ortiz, R. & Alex, S. (1999). Substance abuse prevention in a multicultural community: A community perspective. In S.B. Kar (Ed.). *Substance abuse prevention: A multicultural perspective* (pp.261-269). Amityville, NY: Baywood Publishing Co., Inc.

McGovern. T.F. & White, W.L. (Eds.). (2002). *Alcohol problems in the United States: Twenty years of treatment perspective*. New York: Haworth Press.

Rodriguez-Andrew, S. (1998). Alcohol use and abuse among Latinos: Issues and examples of culturally competent services. *Alcoholism Treatment Quarterly*, 16, pp.55-70.

# Index

AA. *See* Alcoholics Anonymous (AA)
Acculturation, 170
Acculturation Rating Scale for Mexican Americans (ARSMA-II), 174,175
Addiction Severity Index, 154
Adolescent(s)
  Dominican, alcohol use among, 61
  high-risk, substance abuse among
    introduction to, 166-167
    literature review of, 167-169
    prevention of, 165-184
      background in, 171-173
      extant prevention programs in, 169-171
  Latino, high-risk, alcohol/drug use among, onset of, 70-72
Age, of Latino population, 15
Alcohol and other drug (AOD) abuse, religion and, relationship between, 187-189
Alcohol and other drug (AOD) use, among high-risk youth, 165-184. *See also* Adolescent(s), high-risk, substance abuse among
Alcohol services, for Latinos, 206-207
Alcohol Use Disorders Identification Test, 59
Alcohol use/abuse
  among adult Puerto Rican injection drug users, 149-164. *See also* Puerto Rican injection drug users, adult, alcohol use among

among Dominican-Americans, 53-65. *See also* Dominican-Americans, alcohol use among
among high-risk adolescents, prevention of, 165-184. *See also* Adolescent(s), high-risk, substance abuse among, prevention of
among Latinas, incarcerations due to, 87-106. *See also* Latina(s), incarcerated; Latina(s), incarceration of
among Latinos, introduction to, 1-7
children of parents with, rural Latino grandparents raising, 107-130. *See also* Grandparent(s), rural Latino, raising grandchildren of alcohol and drug abusing parents
as factor in Latino population, 16-19
*Alcohol Use/Abuse Among Latinos: Issues and Examples of Culturally Competent Services,* 2
Alcoholics Anonymous (AA), 46,133
Alcohol-related problems, among Mexican-origin adults in central California, 29-51. *See also* Mexican-origin adults, in central California, alcohol problems of
Alcohol-related services, for Latinos, 9-27

# BOOK ORDER FORM!

Order a copy of this book with this form or online at:
http://www.haworthpress.com/store/product.asp?sku=5611

## Latinos and Alcohol Use/Abuse Revisited

*Advances and Challenges for Prevention and Treatment Programs*

―――― in softbound at $24.95 ISBN-13: 978-0-7890-2926-3 / ISBN-10: 0-7890-2926-X.
―――― in hardbound at $39.95 ISBN-13: 978-0-7890-2925-6 / ISBN-10: 0-7890-2925-1.

| | |
|---|---|
| **COST OF BOOKS** _____ | ❏**BILL ME LATER:** |
| | Bill-me option is good on US/Canada/ |
| **POSTAGE & HANDLING** _____ | Mexico orders only; not good to jobbers, |
| US: $4.00 for first book & $1.50 | wholesalers, or subscription agencies. |
| for each additional book | |
| Outside US: $5.00 for first book | ❏**Signature** _____ |
| & $2.00 for each additional book. | |
| | ❏**Payment Enclosed: $** _____ |
| **SUBTOTAL** _____ | ❏ **PLEASE CHARGE TO MY CREDIT CARD:** |
| In Canada: add 7% GST. _____ | |
| | ❏Visa ❏MasterCard ❏AmEx ❏Discover |
| **STATE TAX** _____ | ❏Diner's Club ❏Eurocard ❏JCB |
| CA, IL, IN, MN, NJ, NY, OH, PA & SD residents | **Account #**_____ |
| please add appropriate local sales tax. | |
| **FINAL TOTAL** _____ | **Exp Date** _____ |
| If paying in Canadian funds, convert | |
| using the current exchange rate, | **Signature**_____ |
| UNESCO coupons welcome. | *(Prices in US dollars and subject to change without notice.)* |

**PLEASE PRINT ALL INFORMATION OR ATTACH YOUR BUSINESS CARD**

| | | |
|---|---|---|
| Name | | |
| Address | | |
| City | State/Province | Zip/Postal Code |
| Country | | |
| Tel | | Fax |
| E-Mail | | |

May we use your e-mail address for confirmations and other types of information? ❏Yes ❏No We appreciate receiving
your e-mail address. Haworth would like to e-mail special discount offers to you, as a preferred customer.
**We will never share, rent, or exchange your e-mail address.** We regard such actions as an invasion of your privacy.

Order from your **local bookstore** or directly from
**The Haworth Press, Inc.** 10 Alice Street, Binghamton, New York 13904-1580 • USA
Call our toll-free number (1-800-429-6784) / Outside US/Canada: (607) 722-5857
Fax: 1-800-895-0582 / Outside US/Canada: (607) 771-0012
E-mail your order to us: orders@haworthpress.com

**For orders outside US and Canada,** you may wish to order through your local
sales representative, distributor, or bookseller.
For information, see http://haworthpress.com/distributors

*(Discounts are available for individual orders in US and Canada only, not booksellers/distributors.)*

**Please photocopy this form for your personal use.**
www.HaworthPress.com

BOF05

For Product Safety Concerns and Information please contact our EU
representative GPSR@taylorandfrancis.com Taylor & Francis Verlag GmbH,
Kaufingerstraße 24, 80331 München, Germany

Printed and bound by CPI Group (UK) Ltd, Croydon, CR0 4YY
08/06/2025
01896991-0010